W9-BIQ-159

THE
EVERYTHING
PREGNANCY
BOOK

What every woman needs to know—month-by-month— to insure a worry-free pregnancy

Maryann Brinley

with

Howard Berk, M.D.

Adams Media Corporation
Holbrook, Massachusetts

Copyright ©1999, Adams Media Corporation.
All rights reserved. This book, or parts thereof, may not be
reproduced in any form without permission from the publisher; exceptions are
made for brief excerpts used in published reviews.

An Everything® Series Book.
Everything® is a registered trademark of Adams Media Corporation.

Published by Adams Media Corporation
260 Center Street, Holbrook, MA 02343

ISBN: 1-58062-146-5

Printed in the United States of America.

J I H G F E D

Library of Congress Cataloging-in-Publication Data
Brinley, Maryann Bucknum.
The everything pregnancy book / by Maryann Brinley : introduction by Howard Berk.
        p.   cm.
Includes bibliographical references and index.
ISBN 1-58062-146-5
1. Pregnancy—Popular works. 2. Childbirth—Popular works. I. Title.
        RG525.B666   1999
        618.2'4—dc21   99-11862
                CIP

Many of the designations used by manufacturers and sellers to distinguish their products are claimed
as trademarks. Where those designations appear in this book and Adams Media was aware of a
trademark claim, the designations have been printed in initial capital letters.

The Everything® Pregnancy Book does not purport to render medical advice. Every pregnant woman
should consult her professional health care provider for such advice.

Illustrations by Barry Littmann

This book is available at quantity discounts for bulk purchases.
For information, call 1-800-872-5627 (in Massachusetts, call 781-767-8100).

Visit our home page at http://www.adamsmedia.com

Contents

Month One / 21

Month Two / 43

CONTENTS

Month Four / 107

CONTENTS

Month Five / 127

Month Six / 147

Month Seven / 167

Month Eight / 193

Month Nine / 209

CONTENTS

Introduction

By Howard Berk, M.D.

Women are wonderful patients. I chose obstetrics and gynecology as a medical specialty because it was a combination of medicine and surgery. I was torn between my love for both when I was a young practitioner and obstetrics and gynecology would give me the best of both worlds. The long, unpredictable hours demanded of an OB/GYN did send me straight back to my family for their input. Yet, once everyone said, "Okay," I was certain that this was the perfect medical practice for me.

Over the years, I have been given tremendous opportunities to deal with women under stress. How are they? Terrific. Women are better patients than men. Difficult to take care of, men don't listen and panic at the smallest thing. Meanwhile, women calmly seek answers and information constantly. Some even build personal libraries of books on topics like pregnancy.

There is a joke that I tell every once in awhile, which should make all the women who have picked up this book smile. It's biblical but not preachy. Eve was walking in the Garden of Eden and said to God, "I'd like someone to keep me company. I'm lonely." So, God replied, "Okay Eve, I'll give you a man but you'll have one big problem." Eve inquired, "What's the problem?" Then, God explained, "You'll have to convince the man that I brought you onto the earth first."

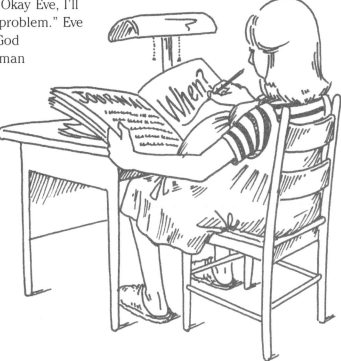

Years ago, I worked on a book with Carole Spearin McCauley titled *Pregnancy After 35*. I enjoyed that experience and consider it a privilege to be involved in a publishing venture once again. Warm, informative, supportive, *The Everything®️ Pregnancy Book* will help readers like you feel right at home throughout your pregnancy, during labor, birth and delivery as well as later on, when you are in your role of brand new mother and definitely need a good friend.

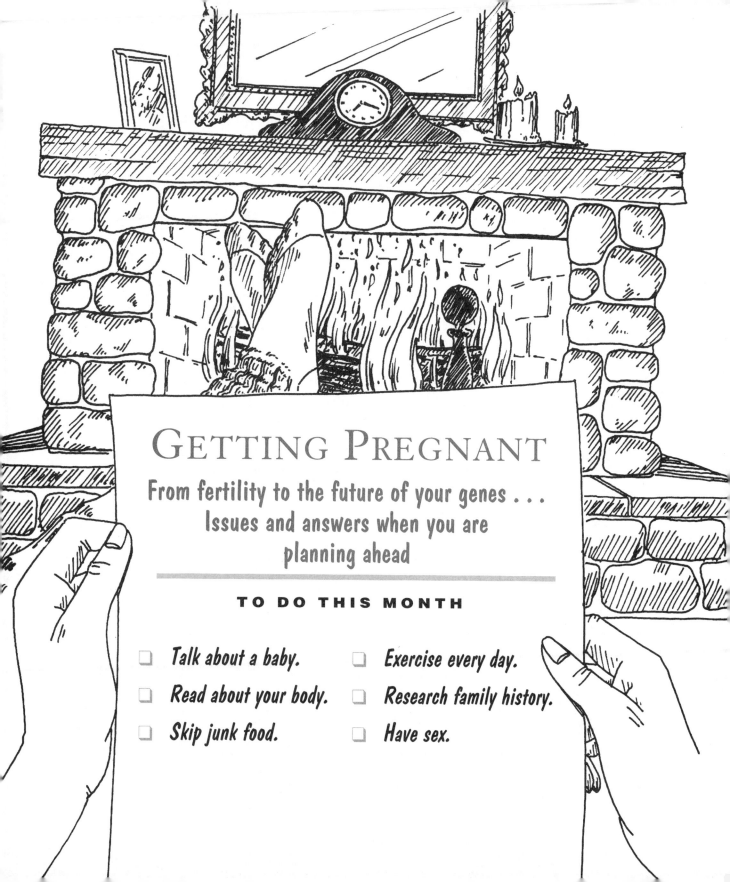

GETTING PREGNANT

From fertility to the future of your genes . . .
Issues and answers when you are
planning ahead

TO DO THIS MONTH

- ☐ Talk about a baby.
- ☐ Read about your body.
- ☐ Skip junk food.
- ☐ Exercise every day.
- ☐ Research family history.
- ☐ Have sex.

From prepartum anxiety to postpartum blues, there is no doubt about it and no need to hide it: Pregnancy can make you feel downright crazy at times. In fact, under old English law, the eccentricity of an expectant mother was once thought to be so serious that her testimony was not considered reliable enough for a court of law.

Relax. You aren't crazy. You are just pregnant . . . or trying to get pregnant! This emotional roller-coaster ride can skew your view of the world. Get ready for confusion, ecstasy, tears, pain, panic, wonder, awe, joy, worry, and a mountain of excessive guilt. Rest assured that you don't need to feel alone on this trip. Moreover, talking about your fears and finding answers to your questions are excellent ideas. No worry is ever too silly to overlook and no question is too stupid to ask.

To calm your fears, put the changes in your life into perspective, and tackle thousands of those "What if" questions swirling just below the surface of your anxiety, start turning the pages. Don't try to read from cover to cover. Flip through sections and find the month, the issue, the symptom, the stage, or the feature that suits your needs right now. *The Everything Pregnancy Book* is designed to be user-friendly. Meanwhile, I'm certain you have a private list of "What if's" already. In fact, the true extent of "what if" nightmares before, during, and after pregnancy can easily fill an encyclopedia. What if I waited too long to try to get pregnant? What if I'm not a good mother? What if my husband's lack of interest in babies now is a predictor of his future success as a father? What if that wine I drank harms my unborn baby? What if I catch toxoplasmosis from my cat? What if my baby isn't normal? What if I flunk Lamaze classes? What if I don't have enough money, patience, or love?

On Your Mark, Get Set, Get Answers

Talking about a baby is so very important for your relationship with the man in your life. Not only do you want to make sure your image of living happily ever after with a family coincides with the picture in his mind, but also you don't want to make the mistake of thinking a baby will cement your partnership. Having a baby to strengthen a relationship is definitely a mistake. Becoming a parent is emotionally and physically hard work. In the best of all possible worlds, both you and your partner ought to begin with your eyes open.

Research Family Histories, Both Yours and Your Mate's

Aunt Edna's red hair, Uncle Albert's big nose, your mother's diabetes, and your father-in-law's hemophilia are suddenly becoming more important. While the red hair and prominent nose may not be of primary concern to you, certain disorders or conditions can be inherited and you will want to know all about them. Diabetes, hypertension (high blood pressure), thalassemia, Tay-Sachs disease, sickle-cell anemia, hemophilia, muscular dystrophy, cystic fibrosis, Huntington's chorea, chromosomal abnormalities, and even twins run in families. Concerned or aware of a family medical issue? Schedule a preconception counseling appointment with your primary care physician. Then, if necessary, a session with a geneticist can clear up any confusion about familial disorders. What's more, you may walk out with a prescription for prenatal vitamins even though you are still getting ready to get pregnant. Ask your family practitioner for a recommendation.

Consider Your Own Health

If you have a long-standing medical condition, make an appointment with your specialist and explain your plans to become pregnant. If you haven't had German measles or toxoplasmosis or you aren't sure, have a blood test to check and get vaccinated before you become pregnant. German measles, especially during early pregnancy, can cause birth defects.

Is your weight average for your height? Being underweight can affect your ability to get pregnant. If you are overweight, now is *not* the time to start a reducing diet. Your unborn baby needs vital nutrients and you are the supplier. You can't hire someone else to supply vitamins, minerals, proteins, and carbohydrates. You're it. If you smoke cigarettes, quit. Drinking alcohol or taking recreational drugs are not good ideas, either. Meanwhile, aerobic exercise (walking or swimming) is just great.

Now, Are You Fertile?

If you have never been pregnant before, you've probably taken your fertility for granted. And why not! What could be more natural! You were born with more than 250,000 follicles or capsules containing immature oocytes, or eggs. Each one of these little eggs is quite capable of turning into your dream baby. Yet, timing is everything in the game of fertility, both in years and in days of your menstrual cycle. The older you get, the less fertile you become. If you are in your twenties, your timing is just right as far as age is concerned. If you are under eighteen, you run a greater risk of having a stillborn or small baby, and if you are over thirty-five, the risks of a difficult pregnancy or of chromosomal abnormalities in the fetus increase. Timing also plays a critical role when you begin to build your sexual life around the days of the month made perfect for reproductive intercourse.

What Makes You Fertile?

To be fertile one of your two ovaries must produce and then release a ripe, healthy egg approximately fourteen days before your next expected period begins. This little egg, or *ovum*, will remain viable for about two days in your reproductive tract. The next thing that must happen depends on your fallopian tubes. You have two tubes, but only one is needed to pick up the ovum as it drops from your ovary or to retrieve it from the floor of your pelvic cavity. The tube must be open, however. Fertilization will take place when healthy sperm enter your vagina and swim upstream through your cervix and uterus and right on into the fallopian tube, which has captured the ovum. One little sperm, only one-thousandth of an inch long, is all that you need to get pregnant. However, this sperm must be strong enough to swim a distance that some experts liken to crossing the English Channel three times without stopping. As it happens, millions of sperm do start the race, but only a few hundred survive this long-distance event and only one will penetrate the egg. The successful sperm manages to strike the egg at just the right angle for penetration. If you could view the process under a microscope, you might actually see the losing sperm battling for entry on the surface of the egg. *Capacitation* is the process by which the sperm actually penetrates the

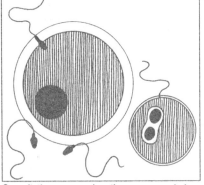

Capacitation occurs when the sperm penetrates the egg (left).

egg, and only sperm that have spent some time in a female reproductive tract, within the egg's environment, have such power. Through a process known as the *acrosome reaction*, the little sperm receives a "stocking cap" on its head, which helps it to release enzymes to create a hole in the egg and, thus, make conception possible. After this happens, the fertilized egg will move down the fallopian tube and on into your uterus, or womb, where it will be implanted in the spongy wall called the *endometrium*. Voila! This is the very point at which pregnancy begins.

Meanwhile, you may be wondering, "Is all this moving, maneuvering for position, egg and sperm orchestration really going to happen inside me?" Yes, at least in the best of all circumstances it will. If all the organs in your reproductive tract are healthy and hormonal factors work in perfect timing, your brain really is the power behind the entire pregnancy process. Your brain signals when some hormones should rush into action and when they ought to slow up. Your emotions, you see, are directly involved with your fertility. In fact, what might seem to be a simple human endeavor—having sex and getting pregnant—soon appears to be more like a miraculous chain of events.

Eight Important Ingredients in Making a Baby

1. Your mate's testicles have to be producing healthy sperm that can swim the distance to your egg and then penetrate it.
2. Your ovaries must be making healthy eggs that are released when you ovulate once a month.
3. To produce the best sperm that are ready to make the long-distance swim up through your reproductive tract, have fun.
4. The egg, which is released when you ovulate, has to be able to make an easy journey to one of your fallopian tubes. Obstructions in the tube, for instance, will interfere with your fertility.
5. Your partner's sperm have to be able to swim freely. If they encounter physical, chemical, or mucus barriers in your cervix, the race toward conception can be lost.

Did You Know . . .

- You were born with more than 250,000 follicles containing immature oocytes or eggs?
- You are more likely to conceive on the thirteenth, fourteenth, and fifteenth days before your next period?
- Seventy-five percent of all couples get pregnant easily within the first six months of trying?

6. After fertilization, your egg has to move to your uterus at a time in your physiological cycle when it can safely implant itself in the uterine wall.
7. The ovum has only twelve to twenty-four hours of life in which to match up with the right sperm.
8. Meanwhile, sperm have twenty-four to seventy-two hours of meaningful life inside your body.

In other words, you and your mate have about three really perfect days during each menstrual cycle to make a baby. The unfertilized egg can live for up to twenty-four hours once a month. If sexual intercourse doesn't take place exactly on target, when both egg and sperm are ready, nothing will happen. So start synchronizing your calendars!

Should You Worry About Infertility?

Probably not. Statistics indicate that 75 percent of all couples can get pregnant easily within the first six months of trying and up to 90 percent will be successful within a year. If you've just begun to consider pregnancy, then don't worry yet. Every day in the world, hundreds of thousands of babies are being conceived.

Body Basics

You can certainly get pregnant without a Ph.D. in human physiology, but sometimes it's nice to know what's in your reproductive tract. Here are just a few basics to help you gain more respect for the organs that are instrumental in pregnancy.

Your Cervix

In Latin, *cervix* actually means "neck," and it's easy to see the origin of this name. Located at the neck of your uterus, your cervix is only about an inch wide but its opening is even smaller so it can protect your uterus from germs or other unwanted invaders. Connected to your uterus, your cervix opens mid-cycle and the reason it opens mid-cycle is that nature has created a wonderful pattern. When you ovulate, the cervix gets larger and the cervical

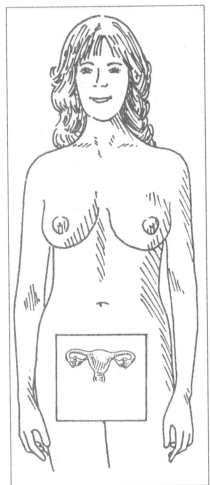

Position of the womb before fertilization.

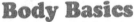

mucus changes. You may notice a mucus discharge in the middle of your menstrual cycle when this mucus consistency changes. Before and after this time, the cervical mucus is thick and viscous to keep your system closed. Only at the time of ovulation, does your cervix dilate and the mucus change so that the sperm can get through. During labor and then delivery, the cervix goes through dramatic changes as it opens to a full ten centimeters, or four inches, to give your baby an opening to the outside world.

Your Vagina

A muscular passage only about four or five inches in length, your vagina is connected to the cervix on the inside and leads to the outside of your body. Most of the time, your vaginal walls stay close together; but during sex, as well as in childbirth, this organ exhibits amazing capabilities.

Your Ovaries

Sitting right within reach of your fallopian tubes are the two little, yellowish walnut-shaped glands known as ovaries. Their color inside your body is unlike nearby structures, which are covered in a greyish protective film. These yellow glands are able to release the eggs they produce monthly as well as the hormones you need to menstruate and to get pregnant. The hypothalamus is an area of your brain that secretes releasing factors. The hypothalamus first secretes follicle stimulating hormone (FSH), which ripens an egg and produces estrogen. When the estrogen gets to a particular level in your body, not only does it turn down the FSH but it causes the release of luteinizing hormone (LH). When the LH comes out, on about the twelfth day, you ovulate. Then, in the ovary, a body forms called the corpus luteum, which maintains the progesterone. If there is no pregnancy, then the corpus luteum fades. Then, you get your period. This is the basic cycle that can happen. All of these messages start from the very beginning of your cycle and not just at the time you are ovulating.

Each month, several eggs will begin to ripen and move, but usually only one rises all the way to the surface of an ovary. If you

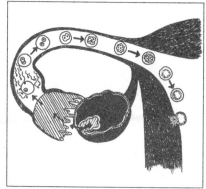

The sperm and fertilized egg follow a distinct path along the fallopian tubes on the way to the uterus.

could get a closer look inside, you would be able to see a lot of uneven pits and bumps on the ovaries, which indicate where other follicles degenerated. In a healthy woman, scars are actually visible, along with stains, from all the monthly activity. For most women, ovulation takes place approximately two to three days following the elevation of LH levels.

How to Figure Out When You Are Ovulating

Having a monthly period is not really an indication of your fertility. Ovulation is the key. Some women have no trouble recognizing exactly when they are ovulating and even feel a twinge of pain on one or the other side of their lower backs in mid-cycle. This is called *mittelschmerz*. Others find the whole process a bit more mysterious. Meanwhile, some conditions can interfere with ovulation without your being aware of the problem even if you are having regular monthly periods. In fact, experts often recommend that you get a clearer picture of your ovulatory cycle if you have been trying to get pregnant for more than six months with no success. One of the first and most basic techniques is to track your *basal body temperature*. Start by planning to take and record your temperature every morning at the same time. An ordinary thermometer is just fine. However, a basal thermometer might make the process easier because it measures only between 96 and 100 degrees Fahrenheit. Have a calendar or date book that you can keep near your bed. Jot down your temperature daily. Your doctor may also be able to furnish you with a special basal body temperature chart. Begin your temperature adventure on the first day of your menstrual cycle, which is the first day you begin to bleed. Take your temperature before you do anything else each morning, even before you climb out of bed. Don't eat, drink a cup of coffee, stand up, or start your exercise program. In fact, the very word *basal* simply means "body at total rest." So don't jump up to grab the thermometer. Take a slow, easy-does-it approach to the process. Before ovulation, the average woman's temperature is 97.5 degrees Fahrenheit. When you are ovulating, this figure may dip a little or remain steady. However, a day or two after ovulation, your temperature ought to rise at least one degree to 98.5 degrees

Fahrenheit, where it will stay until you are about to start your period again. Ovulation is believed to occur within one to two days before your temperature rises. If you notice a change in temperature, jot down possible excuses for the swings, such as exhaustion, illness, or alcohol. If you can stick with this record-keeping for at least three cycles, you will have a much better idea of exactly when you are ovulating and exactly when you are most likely to conceive a baby.

Checking your cervical mucus is another way to gauge your fertility or when you are ovulating. Immediately following your monthly period, hardly any mucus is apparent. In the middle of your cycle, however, mucus will start to be plentiful and sticky. Try inserting your index finger into your vagina to withdraw some for a little test. Is it clear, thin, with the consistency of uncooked egg white? If so, this change indicates the presence of estrogen building up. When you are ovulating, your mucus should be so stretchy that you can pull it apart between your fingers. You may even recall feeling damp or wet during these regular periods of ovulation. If you are trying to get pregnant, copious, stretchy mucus is one of the best signs possible. Make time to make love.

Another way to check for ovulation is to purchase an *ovulation predictor kit* at your nearest drug store. Each home kit features a packet of chemically prepared sticks that test for signs of certain hormonal changes in your urine. As you get closer to ovulation, your body has more luteinizing hormone (LH). After urinating into a small cup, you insert one of the sticks early each morning. Changes in your hormone levels will be reflected in the color that comes up on the stick, anything from white to pale blue to a dark blue, which indicates that you are very close to ovulation. When you see the darkest, bluest color, it's time to have intercourse.

Your Fallopian Tubes

You may know that you have two of them, but perhaps their size—four inches long—and their consistency will come as a surprise. Your fallopian tubes remind some experts of stretched tubes of cooked pasta. Lying just above your ovaries, fallopian tubes have featherlike fingers at the ends closest to the ovaries. They look a

Do You Need to Be "Missionary" Lovers?

While once considered critical, lovemaking positions don't turn out to be as important as actually being together and achieving orgasm. Old stories about the missionary position, with the man on top and the woman lying passively still, aren't going to guarantee a pregnancy. The sperm will know where to go naturally and you don't need to lie on your back for up to a half hour after having sex. Don't worry about any semen leaking out either. It's normal to lose some of the ejaculate after intercourse. What researchers have found, however, is that men are able to produce better ejaculate during the real intensity of intercourse than they are during infertility treatments when forced to masturbate to produce a semen sample.

little like pieces of seaweed floating on the ocean. The little feather tips are called *fimbria*, which is the Latin word for fringes, and they make it easier for the tubes to stretch out and capture the ripened egg at ovulation time. Picture millions of tiny hairs and you'll be able to envision the fimbria better. Mucus and fluids help move the egg into and down the pastalike tube where it waits to meet the sperm. If no suitor appears on time, the egg is simply absorbed back into your body.

Never sell those fallopian tubes short! Lined with muscular ligaments, they actually contract to help sperm and egg move closer together and toward conception. Closer to the uterus, they tighten up to hold onto an egg until the uterus is ready for the planting process, which won't occur until five to seven days after ovulation.

Every once in a while, fallopian tubes are unable to catch eggs as they are released. However, if an egg falls to the floor of your pelvis, fallopian tubes have the power to reach down and pick it up, pushing the egg along closer to conception.

Your Uterus

A hollow organ, the uterus is shaped like a pear and is normally about three inches long. The lining of your uterus, known as the *endometrium*, is velvety and rich in bloody tissue. Sitting right in the middle of your reproductive organs, the uterus, or womb, can hold only about a teaspoon of liquid ordinarily. When you are pregnant, it expands to the size of a watermelon to hold your growing baby, the amniotic fluid, and the placenta. Continually being renewed, the lining of your uterus builds up in response to messages sent by your hormones and then sheds itself once a month during your menstrual period when you don't get pregnant. During the first half of your menstrual cycle, estrogen makes your endometrial lining thicken. As your ovaries release eggs midway through your monthly cycle, progesterone takes over and helps your body get ready for a possible pregnancy. If no fertilized egg finds its way to your womb, the endometrium falls apart and you have a period. Your hormone levels are at their lowest during that very first day of your period.

Ectopic Pregnancy: Bleeding, Pain, and a Positive Pregnancy Test

When the fertilized egg doesn't travel all the way to the uterus for implantation in the endometrial lining, the result can be what is called an ectopic pregnancy. Trying to grow outside the womb, this wayward egg can end up in your abdominal cavity, your ovary, and even on your cervix; but most ectopic pregnancies occur in a fallopian tube. This is why they are often referred to as tubal pregnancies.

A dangerous and potentially life-threatening situation, an ectopic pregnancy will give you warning signs of trouble. The three most important signs, according to New York obstetrician-gynecologist Howard Berk, M.D. are: "Bleeding, pain, and a positive pregnancy test." You may experience severe cramps that begin on one side of your abdomen and travel to the other. This is a sharp, stabbing pain and it may hurt to move. You may start to bleed, be nauseous, dizzy, fatigued beyond the ordinary and you must seek emergency medical treatment immediately. Go to a hospital. Don't wait for the pain to pass. If the fertilized egg ruptures in your fallopian tube, you may bleed throughout your abdominal cavity. Surgery might be scheduled immediately. However, ultrasound and blood tests nowadays can help determine the diagnosis of an ectopic pregnancy. New technology has given practitioners a variety of warning signs so the large majority are detected before they reach crisis proportions.

What Can Cause Infertility?

The actual infertility rate is 12 percent, which means that 88 percent of all couples are fertile.

Yet, a variety of factors can make it difficult for you to get pregnant. Some roadblocks can be easy to correct. Discuss your worries with your doctor or health-care provider and don't wait too long to bring up your concerns. Infertility can be caused by a combination of things: from unexplained factors to ovulatory failure, tubal damage, semen factors, endometriosis, cervical problems, or a hormonal deficiency. When the problem isn't obvious, hormonal and metabolic imbalances could be at fault. Some experts suspect that dietary habits can also cause infertility.

For More Information

For more information regarding infertility, you can contact the American Society for Reproductive Medicine, 1209 Montgomery Highway, Birmingham, AL 35216-2809, phone: 205-978-5000, fax: 205-978-5005, Internet address: http://asrm.org.

Your fertility begins to decline after your thirty-fifth birthday and definitely declines after the fortieth birthday. After your forty-fifth birthday, the reason your periods become irregular is that your fertility has declined even further. If you have an oddly shaped uterus or abnormal growths along your reproductive tract, any slight mismatch of movements between the fallopian tubes and your ovaries can cause infertility. If you've been exposed to dangerous chemicals, certain X-rays, or have a hormonal imbalance, these can also make getting pregnant a problem. Infections and sexually transmitted diseases are also factors in infertility. For example, if you have a history of pelvic infections, your chances of ending up with troublesome scar tissue is greater, and so is your risk of tubal pregnancy, a life-threatening condition.

Intrauterine devices (IUDs) can cause infections and affect your ability to get pregnant. Fluctuations in hormones, genetic factors, and even body fat all play a role. Although it may be considered in style to be thin, if your body fat falls below 17 percent of your total weight, pregnancy can become a tricky matter.

Smoking cigarettes is definitely a habit you want to kick if you are trying to get pregnant. The nicotine in tobacco affects your physiology and high levels have even been found in the cervical mucus of women who smoke. Experts theorize that nicotine can be poisonous to sperm and can change the lining of your fallopian tubes, inflaming them and making them less likely to help in the process of conception.

Quick Tips for Getting Pregnant

If you are in the middle of an infertility nightmare, the problem could be complex and warrant extensive investigation with a specialist. However, sometimes getting pregnant is a simpler matter. Here are a few quick tips to make conditions more perfect for pregnancy.

Make Love at the Right Time

Some days of your monthly menstrual cycle are more perfect than others. In fact, you are more likely to conceive on the thirteenth, fourteenth, and fifteenth days before your next period. Mark those days on your calendar and make time for sex without stress. In fact, don't make love for two days beforehand. Your mate's sperm count should be up during this particularly fertile, mid-month time frame.

Adjust Hygiene Habits

Successful sperm are cool. If your mate wears extra tight jeans or underwear, ask him to switch to loose-fitting clothes. In addition, he should keep out of hot tubs, saunas, long hot baths, or whirlpools to keep his supply of sperm cool. If he's a bicyclist, have him speak with his doctor about the latest news on the effect of long rides on circulation in his groin area.

Decrease Caffeine

The scientific evidence is still inconclusive, but some researchers believe that consuming too much caffeine may interfere with ovulation and sperm production.

Eat Sensibly

Now is not the time to start dieting to lose weight. Eat fresh fruits, vegetables, whole grains, and lean proteins. Ask your doctor for recommendations for vitamins. More nutrients are not necessarily better, however. Too many vitamins can be just as bad as not enough. If you have just stopped taking birth control pills, ask your doctor about prenatal supplements, especially your consumption of folic acid, even though you are not technically pregnant yet. Folic acid should be started about three months before a pregnancy because it helps to prevent spinal abnormalities. Of course, you should continue taking it throughout the nine months; but if you are able to start taking folic acid in advance, you are in a position to ensure a better result for your baby. A steady diet of fast food, sweets, or even vegetables alone are also issues to consider. (See Month Five for more information about folate.)

Don't Overdo Your Exercise

If you are fanatical about your exercise routine, you might want to slow down a bit. Regular exercise during pregnancy is perfectly wonderful and usually recommended. However, intense physical workouts have been shown to interfere with ovulation. Speak with a doctor about your habits before you sign up for the New York marathon, for instance.

Learn to Relax

If you sense that others around you are pushing you for more time, more attention, or more work and you are feeling stretched way beyond your inclinations, stop and slow down. Schedule a yoga class. Read a good book. Take time for yourself each day to do something you've always dreamed about. Overprogramming your life with appointments and lists of must-do's will not help you become pregnant and could work against the natural biochemical rhythm your body needs for fertilization.

Should You Have a Baby?

Crucial Questions to Ask Yourself . . . If You Are Wavering, Wondering, Wishing, or Agonizing About Whether to Get Pregnant

My friend Kate is a thirty-four-year-old lawyer who lives and works in Philadelphia. She called me a while back with an urgent request. "Quick. You're a mother. Tell me. Should I have a baby or shouldn't I? I've decided that I must decide now." Kate is a successful career woman; and although she isn't ecstatic about her current position, she has a loving husband, a nifty house, and professionally she is where she dreamed of being when she was in college. The one feather missing from her cap is motherhood. She has, in fact, postponed having a child for so long that the prospect of having a baby leaves her petrified. For Kate, it seems like an impossible and nearly unnatural step to have to take, and the decision has become an enormous burden. Her husband assures her that he will be there for her, but she must make up her own mind.

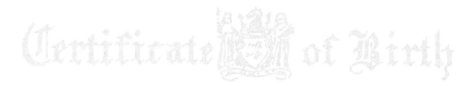

For Your Information:
Food, Glorious Food!

On your pregnancy journey, the sooner you understand the importance of healthy eating, the better you and your baby will be. Experts at the American College of Obstetricians and Gynecologists (ACOG) suggest that a well-balanced diet can speed up conception.

Go for variety, of course, but please include:

- Four or more servings of fruits and vegetables
- Four or more servings of whole-grain or enriched bread and cereal
- Four or more servings of milk and milk products
- Three or more servings of meat, poultry, fish, eggs, nuts, and dried beans or peas

If you've always wondered what nutritionists mean by "serving," here are some guidelines that can help:

- A serving of milk or a milk product is an eight-ounce cup or the equivalent in cheese or any other milk product.
- A serving of bread is a single slice.
- Cereal is one ounce and pasta is one-half to three-quarters of a cup.
- A single piece of fruit is an average serving, but you can also fulfill this requirement by sipping an eight-ounce cup of juice or snacking on a half cup of cooked fruit.
- For protein, two to three ounces of meat, fish, or poultry equal a serving. One egg, three-quarters of a cup of beans or peas, two tablespoons of peanut butter, one-quarter to one-half cup of nuts, sunflower, or sesame seeds will also give you a serving of protein.

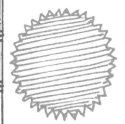

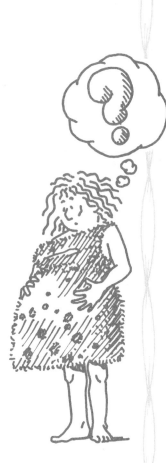

Where are the lists of practical and emotional do's and don'ts, rights and wrongs, for women caught in this bind? When Kate turns fifty, she wants to know, will she envy all the mothers of teenagers? She wonders if she'll become depressed or crazed or lonely as a result of never having exercised her option to have a baby.

She also wonders whether her reasons for wanting a child are all wrong. And, if so, could she have a baby for less than ideal reasons, in imperfect circumstances, and still live happily ever after? Moreover, are there any absolutely right, truly unselfish reasons for having a baby? (After all, how can you be unself-centered in your love for a child during pregnancy, before he or she actually exists—except as an extension of yourself?)

I went looking for answers for Kate and spoke with several professionals who had logical answers. Their wisdom may help you, too.

According to New York psychotherapist Nancy Good, the decision to have a baby always includes some negative and some positive aspects, some wrong and some right reasons, some silly and some sophisticated rationales. Moreover, she says, "any pregnancy begun for what might look like a 'wrong' reason can certainly turn out all right." Dr. Richard Formica, a New Jersey psychologist with experience running workshops for troubled parents, says that shoulds and shouldn'ts abound in this world, "and that's sad. In fact, I hesitate to add more criteria to this very personal, very important decision. But there are considerations anyone can use to examine her readiness for parenthood." The wrong reasons I've listed here aren't absolutely wrong. They are simply guidelines. Having a baby isn't ultimately a checklist proposition.

"Wrong" Reasons to Have a Baby

To Save (or Strengthen) the Relationship with the Man in Your Life

Nancy Good explains that this is still a very common and wrong reason to want a child. "Having a baby out of any kind of fear—especially fear of losing the man in your life—is terribly misguided and may end up backfiring on you. Getting a man to support you or to share his life more with you by having his baby shouldn't be the primary motivating factor in your decision. Sometimes we have emotional needs that did not get satisfied when we were children, and we hope that through a child and a man, we'll make up for this lack. But what's likely to happen is that you'll feel more drained and emptier taking care of a child and a husband. And though you're unhappy with the results, you can't send the baby back to try another tactic."

To Please Your Parents or Your Friends

Other people, no matter how close you may feel to them, are outsiders in your life. They won't be there for the 4:00 A.M. feedings. They may even prove not to be so loving when you don't meet their fantasized expectations of a doting earth mother.

Because Everyone You Know Is Already a Mother

"To consciously choose not to have a child is probably the hardest conditioning a woman may have to overcome in her life," explains Dr. Formica. "When you couple what may be a very real biological drive to reproduce with your need to find your place as a woman, you come up with a pretty powerful force to be reckoned with. But what makes us human is our capacity to experience these drives and not be dominated by them."

To Escape from the Outside Working World

If you have been experiencing frustration in your job and you grew up believing that having a husband and family would bring you automatic self-fulfillment, you may be considering pregnancy as a way out of the outside working world. Don't. Having a baby will not answer all your personal dreams of self-actualization. Moreover, you'll be taking a big step into a new working world where you are required to be on call twenty-four hours a day, seven days a week.

To Squelch a Complete Host of Fears—Once and for All

If you have a child out of fear of being alone in your old age, fear of what you may be missing out on, fear of never winning your mother's approval or your husband's esteem, you may wind up sorry you took the plunge into parenthood.

To Be Loved and Treasured as a Baby Again Yourself

If you haven't put your own childhood behind you, or sorted out the mistakes your mother made from the love she had for you, "then you're not ready to become a mother," insists Atlanta pediatrician Sanford Matthews. In fact, having a baby requires you to grow up.

You've Been Mothering Your Mate and You Think a Real Baby Would Appreciate Your Efforts More

Babies, like some husbands, don't give as much as they take. In fact, as Dr. Matthews says, "If you are looking for the dividends your kids will someday hand you in repayment for your mothering efforts, you're in for a disappointment. Investing your time in diaper changing will never assure you of being able to cash in on dividends down the road. What's more, a husband who has grown pampered and accustomed to uninterrupted doting may have an especially difficult time adjusting to the position of second place in your life."

Your Own Mother Was Not Great at the Task. You Know You Can Do It Better—And Make Up for What You Missed as a Child, Too

"You can't ever make up or remedy the deficits in your own life through your children's," Formica says. "Wanting your children to live for you or do the things you never did is very dangerous." You are robbing your child of her right to a childhood of her own, one that is different from yours and different from the perfect childhood you may envision for her.

To Become Closer to Your Own Mother

Studies have shown that sometimes motherhood can bring a mother and daughter emotionally closer together. But the basis for their togetherness is often a far cry from a state of loving soul sisters. Having a baby to become reunited with your mother may put you right back in the dependent role of daughter instead of that of independent woman.

"Right" Reasons to Have a Baby

I can stand at my kitchen sink, consider Kate's predicament, and know on a very basic, gut level that I made the right decision to have babies. Yet, what can I tell her or you, if you are faced with this very modern dilemma of being able to choose the right time to start a family? Dr. Formica, who was married for thirteen years before starting a family, debated parenthood often with his wife. Here are the seven "right" reasons he and his wife used when they made their decision.

Both You and Your Mate Want and Choose to Have a Child

This is "the most important decision in your life," Formica says, "and you'll be living with the consequences for years. It's much more important than a career choice, so the more explicit and conscious the decision is, the better off you both will be. And I don't believe in compromise on this question of a baby. The wanting is a must for both partners."

Your Aim Is to Give, Rather Than to Get

The idea here, explains Formica, is to want to give "creatively, not sacrificially. Implicit in all sacrificial giving is the heavenly reward or the big payoff later on and that shouldn't be one of your reasons for wanting to give to a child. If problems in your relationship as a couple, or in your life as an individual, are going to prevent you from giving easily to a child, then you may not be ready for parenthood," he explains. "Give because you have something to give and you're going to enjoy the process of giving," he adds.

You Are Going to Give from Your Excess

You aren't going to have that much extra to give if you are still desperately trying to establish yourself in the outside world, if you are still separating from your parents, or if you haven't yet put your act together. But "if you are at that point when you have more than you need, when your life is full to the brim, giving to your own baby can be very rewarding," says Formica.

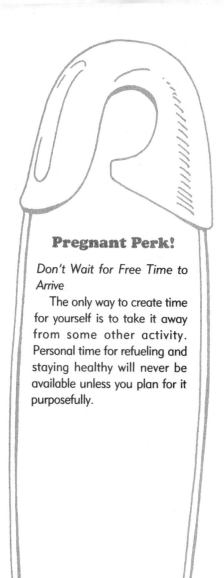

Pregnant Perk!

Don't Wait for Free Time to Arrive

The only way to create time for yourself is to take it away from some other activity. Personal time for refueling and staying healthy will never be available unless you plan for it purposefully.

You Are Going to Be Available, Not Busy

This reason doesn't necessarily call for either parent to stay home with the baby twenty-four hours a day, seven days a week. What it means, says Formica, is "you are not so preoccupied with the external tasks of your life, with developmental goals or career ambitions that you won't be able to spend some 'present' time with your child."

You Want the Challenge of Raising a Child

"In the past," says Formica, "motherhood may have been used as a compensation prize for failure elsewhere in the larger world." But motherhood is not for the weak-hearted, this doctor says, nor is it a retreat from life. So you can't be ready for parenthood until after you have "taken on the challenge of life in the big world."

You're Looking Forward with Pleasurable Anticipation to the Process of Raising a Child

"This is the single most important right reason for having a baby," Formica says. "Rather than looking forward to some narcissistic product that may or may not appear in twenty years, you should be happy to share your life with a child at each stage of his or her life."

You Want to Give Birth to a Personal Expression of Yourself

"You should want to share what you have already made of yourself with your child and not what you hope to become through him or her," Formica explains. "I see this as a very legitimate, healthy form of narcissism. You are saying to yourself and the world, 'I really like me. I like what I am and I want to share my values with a child.'"

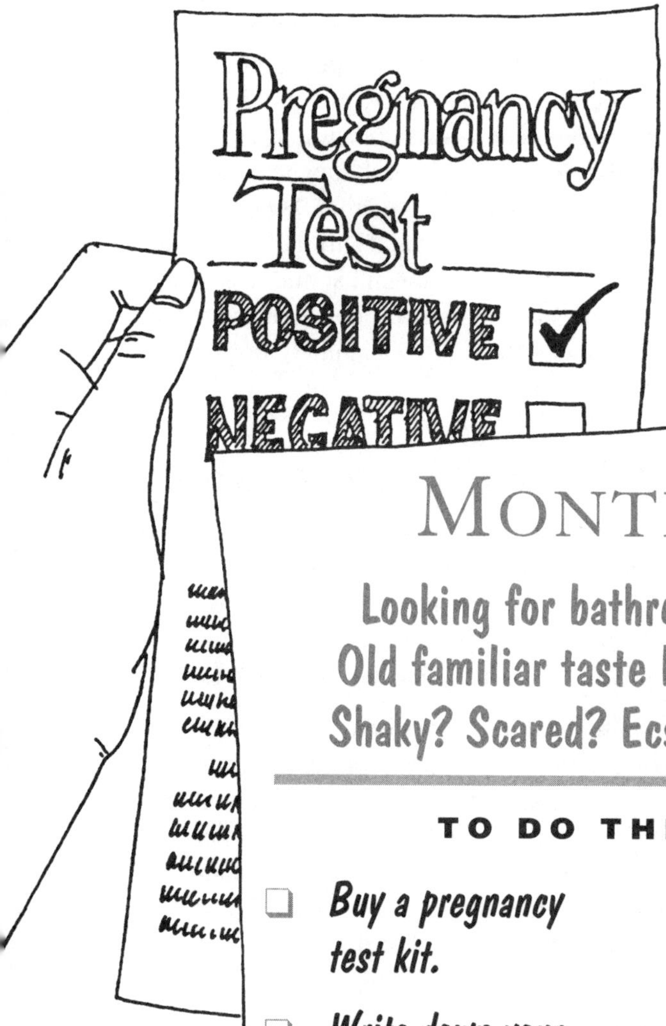

Pregnancy Test

POSITIVE ☑

NEGATIVE ☐

MONTH ONE

Looking for bathrooms everywhere,
Old familiar taste buds gone haywire,
Shaky? Scared? Ecstatic? . . . Happy!

TO DO THIS MONTH

☐ Buy a pregnancy test kit.

☐ Write down your symptoms.

☐ Find a doctor.

☐ Learn about what's happening inside your body.

☐ Figure out your due date.

☐ Get your questions answered.

Whether you are ecstatic about your new state, at the opposite end of the emotional spectrum and feeling blue, or somewhere in between joyful amusement and sheer panic, information is going to be key. In fact, no matter how you feel psychologically, ignorance is never bliss when it comes to pregnancy and childbirth. Changes and challenges are going to come fast.

For most normal women, pregnancy lasts approximately forty weeks, 280 days, nine months or, using childbirth language, three *trimesters* of three months each. Statistics tell us that 95 percent of all babies are born between the 266th and the 294th day after their conception. Two hundred and eighty days doesn't sound like a very long time at all and it isn't, especially when you consider the monumental metamorphosis that your body is now beginning, both physically and emotionally.

What Are You Feeling Emotionally?

Shaky? Scared? Ecstatic? Happy? Nervous? Sick? Energetic? Exhausted? Joyous? Think about it: pregnancy is the only time in your life that you will ever be two people at once! Go easy on yourself.

Oh Baby . . . Inside Secrets Now

Experts are usually uncertain about the exact date of fertilization, so your pregnancy and due date are timed and predicted on the basis of the first day of your last period. However, because unborn life really begins after one of your eggs is fertilized during intercourse, this roughly sketched time line of fetal development and activity is built on that foundation. Some charts of "fetal growth" start back at the first day of your last period and not on the day of fertilization.

- Ovulation occurs around the fourteenth day after your last period and your body releases a healthy egg, ready and able to be impregnated by a successful sperm. Your mate actually ejaculates up to 400 million sperm into your vagina during intercourse, but most never make it to the egg waiting in one of your fallopian tubes. The successful sperm is able to pass

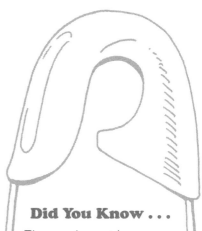

through the soft mucus being secreted by your cervix. If by chance this sperm arrives a little before the egg has been released, it can survive for up to two days.

- Fertilization occurs when the sperm enters the egg, loses its tail, and its head begins to swell. (Swelled head? Right! Sounds like the little guy is proud of his accomplishment!) As this union takes place, a single cell is formed. From this tiny cell, your baby will grow. Although timing the start of a pregnancy is imprecise science, some couples have good hunches about when this new life began based on their sex lives together. Other couples, who have been receiving outside medical intervention for fertility problems, may also have an exact date of fertilization.

- Only a few hours after penetration, the fertilized egg, sometimes called a *zygote*, travels down the fallopian tube toward its destination in the uterus, or womb. It will take six days to reach the uterus and eight to ten days for implantation. As it does so, this cell is dividing, dividing, and dividing again. What you have done is produce a new mixture of chromosomes from both you and your partner. From two cells, there are four. From four cells, there are soon eight, and so on. Some cells divide quicker than others, but as this little fertilized ovum gradually becomes more complicated, it floats down your fallopian tube surrounded by nutrient cells.

- By the end of this first week, a nearly invisible, fertilized ovum may boast anywhere from more than one hundred cells all closely knit into a little ball and ready to move into your uterus. Experts sometimes refer to this fertilized ovum now as a *morula*, which means mulberry in Latin. Inside your womb, the morula finds important nutrients—sugars, salts, and critical elements—for growth. Still floating, it will grow quickly and become more sophisticated as the cells start specializing and taking on different tasks. Some link up to create kidneys. Others complete a small heart to pump blood. Timing is precise and the genetic blueprint, with twenty-three chromosomes from you and twenty-three chromosomes from your mate, lays a course for your unborn baby.

Did You Know . . .

The word *gravida* on your chart doesn't mean *grave* at all but simply *pregnant?*

Just a week after conception, even before you have missed your period, the fertilized egg has twenty-three chromosomes from you and twenty-three from your mate.

- Implantation, or the point at which the fertilized egg attaches itself to the soft, spongy, welcoming lining of your uterus, is now ready to occur. You may be somewhere into your second or third week by now and unaware that such a momentous event is taking place. Some women experience a bit of bleeding when this happens. Little "fingers" or rooting villi from the edges of the fertilized egg reach out to touch you, often on the upper, back wall of the womb. Not only will this ovum develop into your baby, but a few of its rapidly dividing cells will become the placenta that nourishes your baby and the umbilical cord, too, which connects the two of you. You may also hear this fluid-filled cluster of cells referred to as a *blastocyst* now.

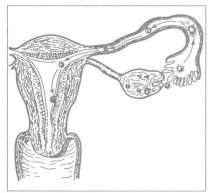

In the first week following conception, the fertilized egg implants in the lining of the uterus.

- If you were to try to picture this happening inside your uterus, imagine a blister. "Implantation looks like a translucent blister on the lining of the uterus," according to noted physician Virginia Apgar. Yet, it's like no blister you've ever experienced in the outside world. As Apgar explained, "The hollow cluster of new cells burrows its way into the lining of the uterus, pushing aside some of the maternal cells and destroying others, tapping into the maternal blood vessels and using maternal blood and cell bits for nourishment." One of the more amazing aspects of this process is that your own body doesn't reject such an invasion, see it as foreign, or try to destroy the little morula, now perhaps the size of the top of a pin. Although your unborn baby's tissues may be very different from yours, your body's immune system doesn't treat them as different. Your biochemistry seems to undergo a dramatic attitude adjustment, accepting the "new kid on the block" peacefully. A bacterial or viral invasion would be a different story indeed. Such peace would never be possible if you weren't pregnant.

- After the first week and up to the eighth week of life, the product of your conception is called an *embryo*. Can you imagine that your own little embryo has a tiny beating heart, which looks like a large bulge at the chest front? A rudimentary brain and spinal cord are also present. Shallow pits on the sides of the head show where eyes and ears will later grow. In size, picture anywhere from one-quarter inch to one and one-tenth inches long.

- At this point, you haven't even missed your period yet. In fact, that rich, spongy lining in your uterus, which served the implantation adventure quite well, is what would have been shed during regular monthly menstruation. Because you have an embryo growing, changing, and manufacturing profound changes in your womb, you miss this monthly event, experiencing one of the first clear signs of pregnancy. The embryo is secreting a hormone, known as human chorionic gonadotropin (HCG), into your blood system, which interferes with menstruation. This is the hormone that will appear in your urine on a pregnancy test and alert you to the news of a new life beginning.

- By the end of the first real lunar month (four weeks) of growth, some of the rapidly dividing cells inside this little "blister" form the placenta, growing more inroads into your uterine cavity and paving the way for its expanding job of nourishing the unborn baby. Inside, the embryo is lengthening and becoming encapsulated in what appears to be a water-tight balloon sac, called the *amnion*. Fluids from your own body fill the sac and cushion your baby from all the bumps, lumps, and movement in your busy life. Known as the amniotic fluid, this watery substance keeps a consistent temperature and provides a weightless environment that allows the developing baby to exercise and move around.

- Next to the embryo another little sac appears. Called the *yolk sac*, this teeny cluster of cells always floats nearby, consists of tiny blood vessels, and provides the blood for the embryo, which is still too immature to do so for itself.

- Other kinds of growth and activity are also taking place during the end of this first month. For example, a third, bubblelike shelter must house the embryo, the amnion, and the yolk sac. On one side of the chorion are numerous little villi that grow into your uterus and form intricate webbings of

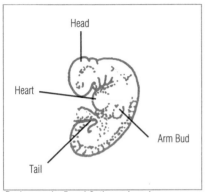

During weeks 5 and 6, the embryo is now ¼-inch, about the size of an apple seed.

blood vessels, multiplying, criss-crossing, and interlocking constantly to feed the placenta and give the embryo everything it could possibly need, including the umbilical cord. Quietly, the frenzy of this one-month production builds. Cells work frantically. You've got a baby in the making.

- Take an imaginary look at your embryo near the very end of this fourth week, and you might be amazed at how very specialized the existing three layers of growing cells have become. From the outer layers will come your baby's nervous system as well as the skin, hair, oil, and sweat glands. Meanwhile, in the middle will form the muscles, bones, kidneys, blood vessels, connective tissues, and even genital glands. Inside, the deepest layer of cells will eventually become important systems such as the digestive, the lungs, and the urinary tract. Early signs of a mouth, face, and throat are in place. Speeding at an incredibly fast pace, the unborn baby's heart, a U-shaped tube that can be seen beneath the opening for the mouth, contracts, perhaps hesitantly at first, but regularly by the end of the fourth week. Beating 180 times a minute, the heart rate starts off very rapidly and through the pregnancy, it declines to about 140 as the baby's system becomes more complex. When you are forming small capillaries, those blood vessels impede the blood so the baby can pick up more oxygen and the heart doesn't have to beat as fast. Pumping blood through the developing systems, this heart may be the clue you are waiting to hear in one of your upcoming doctor's visits.

- Dramatic changes occur almost overnight now. You are officially six weeks pregnant, but your tiny embryo is four weeks along. With no arms visible on days 24, 25, or 26, he or she will produce arm buds within hours and in the speed of just another day, clumps grow into what look like paws, with visible signs of finger growth, too. Leg growth is apparent soon after. Think about it: your body is providing the womb and your baby is growing arms and legs. As Dr. Virginia Apgar stated, "Never again will this human being grow as rapidly or change as much as it has during the first month of prenatal life." Still tiny, of course, your embryo is 10,000 times bigger than he or she was as a fertilized ovum. For a more tangible guide, imagine an apple seed.

Let's Get Physical

Everyone is different, but in the first weeks after conception there are early signs of pregnancy that are quite predictable. Set off by the marked shift in hormone levels in your body, some of these symptoms may disappear after the end of your first three months. Meanwhile, if you think you might be pregnant, watch for these changes:

- You missed your period. If your menstrual cycle is normally irregular, you are under a lot of stress, or feeling sick, this may not be a dependable signal. It is also possible to have a light, bloody discharge and still be pregnant. Some experts say that up to 22 percent of all expectant women report some bleeding early on.
- Your breasts are sore. Tender, enlarged breasts may even tingle and become extra sensitive to touch.
- You are nauseous. Morning sickness, one of the classic signs of pregnancy, doesn't always happen in the morning. You can feel sick at any time of day.
- You are exhausted and sleepy. Falling asleep at your desk? Dreaming of an afternoon nap? Ready for bed at 8:00 P.M.? Fatigue is a predictable signal of early pregnancy.
- You need to urinate frequently.
- You feel faint or a little dizzy.
- You have an achy, heavy sensation in your pelvis.
- You've become intensely emotional. Emotional instability is not all in your head, so don't let anyone try to convince you that you are crazy. Hormonal changes are partly to blame.
- Your taste buds have changed. Some women suddenly develop a strong distaste for alcohol, coffee, and cigarette smoke and complain of a metallic sensation in their mouths. Others begin to crave particular foods.

Soooo . . . Other Pregnant Women Have These Symptoms, Too:

- Tender breasts
- Fatigue
- Occasional dizziness
- Frequent urination
- Nausea
- Insomnia
- Constipation
- Indigestion
- Stomach as well as intestinal gas
- Runny nose
- Headaches
- Signs of varicose veins
- Cravings for strange foods; aversions to old favorites
- Weird changes in skin and hair

Confirm Your Pregnancy

Approximately two weeks after conception or just one day after you miss your period, an obstetrician, nurse-midwife, or clinic practitioner can confirm your pregnancy by testing a sample of your urine and examining you internally. What a pregnancy test is actually measuring is a circulating hormone known as *human chorionic gonadotropin*, or HCG, produced by pregnancy tissues and present in both your blood and your urine after conception. In your grandmother's day, the urine containing HCG was actually injected into a frog or rabbit to uncover a budding pregnancy. Nowadays, doctors have more accurate ways of detecting the level of HCG in your system called immunoassays. However, it is very difficult to detect any pregnancy changes in a uterus one day after a skipped period. Not until implantation has occurred at days 6 through 10, and it is only at that time that hormones are being excreted. So at ten to fourteen days, you can begin to pick up changes and detect a pregnancy.

Home pregnancy kits, which use an immunoassay test, are available in most pharmacies and may be the fastest route to answer this major life question: Are you pregnant? Follow the package directions carefully. Kits rely on a chemical. When combined with your urine in a little test tube, this chemical will change colors in the presence of HCG.

Determine Your Due Date

A very small percentage, 5 percent, of expectant women actually deliver babies on the official due date. Most give birth between thirty-eight and forty-two weeks and are considered full-term. However, first-time moms tend to deliver late. Having a deadline is not only nice but also important. You want to avoid delivering your baby prematurely because of the risk of complications. And, going too long past the due date (a *postterm* or *postdate* pregnancy) can bring other kinds of health risks for you and your baby. The reasons why labor and delivery don't start on time aren't easily understood. Sometimes, a postdate pregnancy has just been a miscalculation of conception. Also, if you've delivered a baby before, you are more likely to deliver within four days of your due date.

Do Your Math

Obstetricians and childbirth specialists have a chart that makes predictions easy, especially if you've always had a regular twenty-eight-day menstrual cycle. However, there are two ways to check for a date on your own by using simple formulas:

- Count 280 days from the first day of your last period. If that day was November 1, for instance, you would pull out your calendar, flip forward through the months and find August 8 to be your due date.
- You can also take that date of your last period, count three months back, and then add seven days. For example, if your last period began on September 1, you would go back through August, July, and into June. Then add seven days to come up with an estimated due date of June 8.

Go Pro . . .

Finding the right medical help to guide you through this very important year of your life is absolutely essential.

- If your gynecologist also practices obstetrics, your search might be over, especially if you are in a high-risk category. A specialist could be important in an emergency.
- Check your health insurance coverage to see if the plan or your managed care company has a list of approved obstetrical practices.
- Your family practitioner can help or may even be able to monitor your pregnancy and deliver your baby.
- Certified nurse-midwives are also an option for some women.

If you don't already have a doctor you trust and with whom you feel comfortable and confident, start investigating now. In fact, buy a large file folder and mark it "Pregnancy." Getting organized so you can collect names, phone numbers, sources, suggestions, pamphlets, and other important items about pregnancy and childbirth could be invaluable. You don't want to spend days looking for that 800 number for free referrals.

To Find the Perfect "Pro"

- Call your county medical society and explain that you want the names of three obstetricians practicing in your geographical area.
- Ask friends, co-workers, neighbors, other doctors for recommendations as well as your health care plan provider. Collect beautiful birth stories so you can create your own dream come true by using the person who helped make everything go so beautifully for other expectant couples.
- Call the nearest hospital or your favorite major medical center and describe your situation. Be specific. For instance, if you think you'd like to have a woman doctor and preferably someone with a midwife on staff, say so. If you've read about the benefits of some aspect of labor and delivery—a birthing room, for instance—ask about it right away. By the way, a hospital's approach to childbirth may even determine the doctor or practice you choose. If you like the hospital, ask about practitioners who have medical privileges established there.
- The American College of Obstetricians and Gynecologists (ACOG) can also provide you with help. Write to their resource center at 409 Twelfth Street, SW, PO Box 96920 Washington, DC 20090-6920. ACOG also operates an Internet Web site at http://acog.com. To find a nurse-midwife, contact the American College of Nurse Midwives, 1522 K Street, NW, Washington, DC 20005, and send a self-addressed, stamped envelope for their reply (Web site: http://www.midwife.org).
- Your local library may have a copy of *The Directory of Medical Specialists*. Each entry features not only the doctor's name and specialty but also where he or she went to school, affiliated hospital, address, phone number, and even age and birthplace.

Essential Ingredients for the First Appointment

When you've narrowed down your choices for a team of professionals to steer your pregnancy, telephone the office, and explain

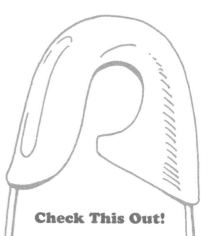

to the nurse or receptionist that you are pregnant and have questions to ask about the practice. Keep in mind that many obstetric, childbirth, and midwifery practices are very busy during patient visiting hours. Don't push for immediate details right there on that first phone call. Ask about a time of day when exploratory calls like yours might be easier to handle. However, listen closely to the tone of voice you hear on your initial telephone connection. Even very busy professionals can demonstrate their potential for kindness. Don't put up with rudeness. You are about to hire someone to help you through one of the most important undertakings of your life.

Do Your Own Research: Getting Answers Upfront

You probably have millions of questions, but here are some that may not be as obvious to you. Write down all your concerns. Don't trust your memory. Once you are under the care of a particular physician or group practice, you'll have lots of question and answer sessions on a regular basis, but a little preliminary research will go a long way toward establishing a wonderful rapport later. You just don't want to be shocked later when you discover something disturbing about your doctor's policy. You are much better off asking upfront. Don't worry about appearing to be too inquisitive. Ask away.

- *How much will it cost?* (Yes, of course money matters.) Check into your health insurance policy to find out how pregnancy is handled. Then, be sure to ask the doctor how much your pregnancy will cost and exactly what the fee includes.
- *Can my husband or friend stay with me during labor and delivery?* This sounds like a concern from the dark ages but you may want to hear the official policy on visitors at these crucial times.
- *Who will deliver my baby?* If the doctor is a sole practitioner, ask about back-up care. You'll want to know the practitioner he or she uses to fill in on vacations, for instance. However,

Check This Out!

Did you know that you can check the credentials of any physician in a specialty by telephoning the American Board of Medical Specialists' hotline: 1-800-776-2378. Obstetricians and gynecologists are specialists who have received extra training and have passed certifying examinations in their area of expertise.

if you are a patient in a group of childbirth professionals, you may want to talk about your need to get to know all the specialists during the nine months so you aren't greeted by a stranger when you go into labor and suddenly get the doctor on call for that particular night or day.

- *Will I be able to move around during labor?* Some experts believe that lying flat on your back during your entire labor can actually slow the process. Perhaps you need to know how the doctor feels about laboring women doing laps through the hospital corridor. (For more about hospitals, birthing centers, and home births, see Month Seven, page 171.)
- *What is your policy on amniocentesis, pain medication, routine fetal monitoring, or drugs to induce labor?*
- *Will I stay in my room to deliver the baby or be moved to a special delivery suite?*
- *How do you feel about episiotomies?* An episiotomy is a cut sometimes made between the vagina and the anus near the very end of labor to help the baby's head pass through. (See Month Nine for more about episiotomies.)
- *How long will I stay in the hospital after the birth?* Some insurance companies also have policies on this question of recuperation time in the hospital. Find out what your plan specifies and ask the doctor if he or she ever intervenes to extend the stay, and what the hospital visiting hours are.
- *Is there a special neonatal unit?* If not, where will any baby who needs extra help be transferred? Though you don't want to anticipate trouble, knowing exactly how the doctor and hospital handle emergencies is important. A neonatal unit can be a very important part of a hospital.
- *What is your approach to weight gain during pregnancy?* Some physicians are known for watching their patients closely and actually trying to manage weight gain. Others take a more laissez faire approach, knowing that in many cases, weight is not easily controlled or predictable during pregnancy.

During a Typical Trip to the Doctor's Office . . .

What can you expect from your regular prenatal trips to the doctor's office? In fact, how often will you find yourself in the offices? Will check-ups differ from your gynecological examinations? Here are answers you need:

If your pregnancy proceeds along without complications, you'll probably have appointments once a month at least for the first seven months of pregnancy. After that, you may be going more often, especially in the last month. The first visit may be one of the longest because it will include a thorough physical exam, complete with blood tests, weight and height checks, and health history. Even if the nurse or receptionist doesn't indicate how long it will take, to be safe, set aside extra time especially if you are taking off from work. You probably have a lot of questions to be answered in this face-to-face session. The doctor will want to know your blood type and he or she will check for the presence of what is known as the rhesus or Rh factor, which can complicate your pregnancy. An internal exam will assure the doctor that your cervix is closed tightly. At this first visit, the issue of any sexually transmitted diseases may come up. Other conditions such as sickle-cell anemia may be discussed. If you've had German measles and can remember when, this will also go on your chart because, though it is a common childhood disease, it can be a problem in pregnancy. Don't forget to ask about prenatal classes or workshops for expectant parents. Some of these classes start early in pregnancy while others may be scheduled later in the third trimester.

When you look at your chart, you will learn new words. Because you are pregnant, you may see the term *gravida*, next to your name. It doesn't mean you are in a grave condition. *Gravida* simply means that you are a pregnant woman. If this is your first baby, you will be called a *primigravida*. *Multigravida* indicates that you have been pregnant before, even if the pregnancy ended in a miscarriage or abortion. *Para*, another

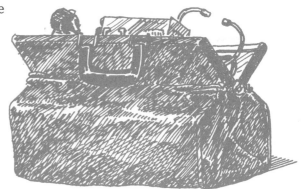

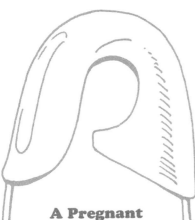

foreign-looking term, means that you delivered a baby past the twentieth week of pregnancy. For instance, you might see *primipara*, which defines a woman who has delivered a baby once before and after the twentieth week.

Check Out Your Check-Ups

You'll be giving urine samples.

At each visit, you will be asked to urinate into a little cup, in private. After showing you to the examination room, asking you to take off your clothes and slip into the gown, the nurse or assistant will routinely hand you a little plastic cup and direct you to the nearest bathroom. Most women have no problem going to the bathroom frequently during pregnancy. Even a small sample is just fine. What your practitioner is looking for are traces of sugar that might indicate that you are developing diabetes. He or she also checks for signs of protein, which is a warning that your kidneys aren't working properly. Late in pregnancy, if the presence of protein is detected, it signals a serious condition called *preeclampsia*, in which your blood pressure rises and you risk suffering convulsions.

Someone will weigh you.

Get ready to gain. Pregnancy weight gain is not always as easily or steadily controlled as expectant mothers or doctors would prefer. The charts say that you should aim for a total gain of twenty-five to thirty pounds evenly added month by month in small increments. However, some women have months of wild growth and others where those numbers on the scale stay pretty steady. Somewhere in my second trimester after fitting the pregnancy textbook gains perfectly, I suddenly went up nearly seven pounds overnight. (Well, if not exactly overnight, I did gain almost instantaneously.)

Your legs, ankles, and hands will be observed to check for swelling.

The doctor or midwife will want to make sure that you aren't retaining fluids, so she or he will check your legs, ankles, or hands.

A Pregnant Pounds Primer

Not all the weight you gain will end up in your baby. Here's how a 25- to 30-pound weight gain breaks down:

- 4–6 lbs basically for you, stored in fat, protein, and other nutrients
- 2–3 lbs of increased fluids in your body
- 3–4 lbs of increased blood volume
- 1–2 lbs for enlarged breasts
- 2 lbs for enlarged uterus
- 6–8 lbs for your baby
- 2 lbs of amniotic fluid
- 1½ lbs of placenta, the tissue connecting you to your unborn baby, which handles all the feeding and cleansing

You'll want to hear the baby's heartbeat.

Not at the first visit, but at all subsequent ones, an electronic device called a fetoscope or a sensitive ultrasound instrument called a Doppler device, will soon let you and your doctor listen to the baby's heartbeat. Those first sounds of your unborn baby's heartbeat may appear near Week 10 but more certainly about Week 12. They are actually the first *real* proof that you are pregnant. Don't miss any opportunity to lend your own ear to the event. Later, after Week 18 to 20, a standard stethoscope will pick up the beat.

Your abdomen will be poked, prodded, and measured.

To check the position of the womb at each stage, you may look forward to this step at every appointment. (For more advance warnings about what might be in your doctor's bag of tools and tests, turn ahead to Month Three.)

I Was Wondering . . .

Is there anything my husband and I may have done that might influence our baby's sex?

Although men don't always want to know this, they hold the key to the baby's sex, not you. Men have two different kinds of sperm, male and female. Back in the 1960s, a doctor named Landrum B. Shettles discovered that he could tell the difference between these two types of sperm. Males were supposedly faster than females. Under a microscope, males were also round-headed and appeared to be quite fragile. By contrast, the female sperm had oval-shaped heads and were reputed to swim slower than their male counterparts. However, female sperm were stronger and could last longer even inside a woman's body. Dr. Shettles theorized that to make a boy, you could increase your chances of success by timing intercourse to take place when you were most fertile; appoximately fourteen days after the first day of menstruation. The male sperm would head straight and fast for the ripe egg. To make a girl, you would be better off having intercourse two or three days before you expected to be fertile. Doing it this way, the sturdier female sperm would be more likely to impregnate the egg. Shettles's theories haven't been proven, and in the meantime some experts discounted the whole notion of faster swimming male sperm.

Meanwhile, the most recent research news on choosing the sex of your baby comes from investigators in Fairfax, Virginia, who have been able to presort sperm based on DNA and help couples produce baby girls. Sperm carrying the X chromosome, which creates a female, are actually heavier than those carrying the Y chromosome. Their results, published in the journal *Human Reproduction* and based on a U.S. Department of Agriculture method developed for farm animals, aren't yet perfect but are dramatically close to being accurate in preselecting the sex of a baby. If you are at risk for having a baby with a genetic disease that could be avoided by prechoosing the child's sex, then this new option is good news. A number of genetic disorders affect only males, for instance, and for couples legitimately worried about such outcomes, the Genetics and IVF Institute's fertility research could be most welcome. "There's no question that it works," says Dr. George Seidel, a professor of physiology at Colorado State University. For couples simply trying to balance a family between boys and girls, this new method may not be a reasonable option yet because of the considerable laboratory intervention and expense.

I'm always freaked out by internal gynecological examinations. What exactly is the doctor doing down there now that I know I am pregnant?

There aren't very many women (if any) who relish the idea of internal or pelvic examinations. The doctor or midwife is checking for signs to confirm the fact that you are really pregnant. Like the urine or blood tests, there are objective pieces of evidence that are certainly important:

- *Goodell's sign.* Your vagina and cervix start to retain fluid and actually become softer when you are pregnant.

Ordinarily, your cervix is hard, and as one expert explained, it might even feel like the tip of your nose. After about six weeks of pregnancy, it becomes as soft as your lips. In women who have been pregnant before, this softening may begin even sooner than six weeks.

- *Hegar's sign.* The doctor or midwife inserts two fingers into your vagina in order to touch the uterus. If you are six weeks' pregnant, your uterus will be softer than normal.
- *Chadwick's sign.* The color of your vagina, vulva, and cervix will turn bluish or even violet after two months of pregnancy because of the increased blood congestion and dilation of veins.

Other changes that a skilled childbirth practitioner can see are your enlarging uterus, which begins to change shape from pear like to globular. There will be soft spots on the uterus where the embryo has implanted. Your practitioner may also put his or her fingers across the vagina to feel for signs of throbbing blood vessels.

Are my risks of miscarrying higher because I'm over thirty years old?

With every birthday after your thirtieth, the risks of a miscarriage or spontaneous abortion increase. For women under thirty, some experts predict a 10 percent chance, but this figure escalates to 18 to 20 percent when you turn thirty-five; and after age forty, your chances of losing the baby early in pregnancy are up to three times higher (up to 45 percent). (For more complete information on miscarriage, go to Month Three.)

I'm just so exhausted even though I'm not doing nearly as much as I did before getting pregnant. What's the matter with me?

The level of hormones, estrogen, progesterone, and chorionic gonadotropin rise in your body during these first weeks of preg-

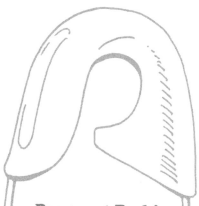

Pregnant Perk!

Allow Yourself Regular Leisure Time

If you think of your time as scarce or as precious money to spend, you will feel fragmented trying to use it wisely. Leisure time is a necessity now, not a reward for having completed everything. Deep benefits for both you and your unborn baby come from forgetting your chores and what time it is. Take a magazine into the bathroom, fill the tub, climb in, and relax. Such a leisurely soak will give you the strength to do more later. Besides, you may not have many opportunities for such a luxury after the baby is born.

nancy and your body needs time to adjust. Progesterone is often blamed as well as the fact that the placenta is still being formed. You actually require more hours of sleep each night when you are pregnant. Remember when you were a teenager and could sleep all Saturday morning long if the people in your life would let you? Well, you need that kind of sleep now. Don't think of yourself as being a slacker. Take a nap. You didn't feel guilty about sleeping late when you were a teen and early pregnancy can demand just as much rest as adolescence. If you can't get to bed earlier at night or sleep late in the morning, plan some naptime. Even a few minutes' rest during the day can reenergize you for hours. Meanwhile, if you are cranky and unable to think straight, don't try to forge ahead during the day. These are signs of exhaustion, so slow down. Your growing baby needs you to be relaxed and well rested.

The weirdest thing has been happening in my mouth for the past three weeks. I can't stop salivating and I wonder if this has anything to do with my pregnancy.

What's happening to you is not weird at all. Known as *ptyalism*, excessive salivation is rare but usually shows up early in pregnancy and can last the entire nine months. Saliva can actually fill your mouth up to the point where you can't avoid spitting. The sour taste can be pretty awful as well. Some experts suggest using mouthwashes, rinsing with water regularly, sucking mints, candies, or lemon slices, brushing your teeth often, and even cutting down on the starches in your diet. Supposedly, starch aggravates the problem. Others suggest eating many small meals during the day and keeping an empty bowl next to your bed for spitting during the night. There are some medicines that can be used to control ptyalism. Consult your doctor about this because there are potent drugs that can be used early in pregnancy.

Should I alter my exercise routine now that I'm pregnant? I walk every day for about forty-five minutes and I've been taking an aerobics class twice a week for years.

It is always important to discuss your exercise routine with your practitioner, but staying in shape during pregnancy is also a great idea. Walking is fine, and your aerobics class may be just as acceptable. The important thing to remember is not to exercise to a point where you are tired or out of breath. Make sure you tell your teacher that you are pregnant. He or she may be able to adjust the regular routine to fit your needs. A certified exercise instructor should know how to trouble shoot for you while you are pregnant. For instance, exercises that pull on the abdominal muscles may have to be avoided. Sit-ups are an example. Jogging may not be well suited to pregnancy, especially in the second and third trimesters, because of the jarring effects of your heels hitting the ground and how stressful the motions can be on your joints and lower back. Speak with your doctor. Describe your athletic history in detail. These nine months are not the time to begin any new fitness craze.

You may be able to keep on doing exactly what you are already doing, but do check it out with a pregnancy expert. Use common sense. For instance, you probably won't want to schedule introductory lessons in skiing, water-skiing, or adventure activities such as mountain climbing or hang gliding. The more physically fit you remain during pregnancy, the faster you will be able to return to your old shape after the baby is born. Exercise is also great for relieving stress and for increasing blood flow to the placenta nourishing your growing fetus. (For more information about exercise routines, see Month Two.)

Could feeling faint be related to my pregnancy?

Yes. Blood pressure is lower when you are pregnant and you are more likely to feel faint. Don't jump up quickly after you've been sitting or lying down. In fact, turn your body to one side when you are climbing out of bed. Anticipate occasions when you know you will

A Doctor's Note: Weight Gain Wisdom

As long as good nutrition remains present and you keep up with all the important vitamins as well as your balanced diet, I have no objection to you trying to control your weight gain during pregnancy. Yet, I don't believe it's necessary to use calories as a guide. Staying active and physically fit is important and keeping up with those vital nutrients. Weight gain is actually a product of genetics, certain diseases, and environmental factors. For example, diabetes increases the weight while hypertension decreases it. Cigarette smoking also decreases the weight. These things have their marked effect. Usually, in utero weights are related to mothers and not to fathers, who only have an influence after birth. What that means is that you will follow in your mother's footsteps. If possible, ask her to recall the weight she gained when she was pregnant with you.

—Howard Berk, M.D.

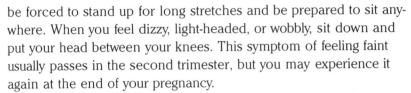

be forced to stand up for long stretches and be prepared to sit any-where. When you feel dizzy, light-headed, or wobbly, sit down and put your head between your knees. This symptom of feeling faint usually passes in the second trimester, but you may experience it again at the end of your pregnancy.

I'm so hungry suddenly. Am I supposed to be eating more than I normally do?

Yes, the National Research Council of the National Academy of Sciences, believes that you need to eat at least 300 more calories a day to support your growing fetus. Think of this as an extra bagel with cream cheese, an additional tuna fish sandwich, or two to two and a half cups of low-fat milk. You don't really need to "eat for two," as the old saying suggested, but your recommended dietary allowances certainly do increase.

Meanwhile, food cravings and aversions to some foods are common. Just because you are ravenous doesn't mean that your body is actually nutritionally deficient. Feel like eating some pickled onions and ice cream? Fine. Just do it. Keep in mind that almost anything you consume when you are expecting a baby can make its way to your baby via the placenta. You are your baby's source of food so if you are craving only salty potato chips, think about adding other nutrients to this wish list. Aim for a variety of fresh, unprocessed foods. Cheeses, milks, and yogurt will give you calcium and proteins. Dark, green leafy vegetables will provide you with vit-amin C, fiber, and folic acid. Lean red meats will give you iron and protein. Liver offers you protein and iron. Oranges can boost your vitamin C quotient and give you fiber, too. Poultry is a good source of protein and iron. Fish such as flounder, tuna, salmon, or bluefish will offer you protein. Hungry right now? Make a peanut butter sand-wich on whole-grain bread.

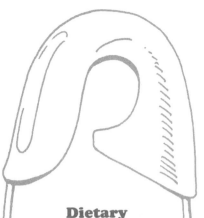

Dietary Requirements During Pregnancy

Here's a chart of exactly how much more you need now that you are pregnant. The percentage refers to the increase over what you used to eat before becoming pregnant:

- Overall Calories = 14% more
- Protein = 20% more
- Vitamin D = 100% more
- Vitamin E = 25% more
- Vitamin K = 8% more
- Vitamin C = 17% more
- Thiamin = 36% more
- Riboflavin = 23% more
- Niacin = 13% more
- Vitamin B6 = 27% more
- Folate = 122% more
- Vitamin B12 = 10% more
- Calcium = 50% more
- Phosphorus = 50% more
- Magnesium = 14% more
- Iron = 100% more
- Zinc = 100% more
- Iodine = 17% more
- Selenium = 18% more

I have become extremely emotional, racing from tears to euphoria. What is wrong with me?

There is nothing wrong with you. Your moodiness is actually referred to as "emotional lability," and it can affect all expectant mothers occasionally or all the time. Are you crying over silly problems? Are you having anxiety attacks? Are you feeling giddy with laughter at inappropriate occasions? Depressed? Confused? Fearful? Your hormones may be affecting your central nervous system, which can make you feel as if you were walking around in a daze. Think about premenstrual syndrome. Were you ever weepy, short-tempered, or irrational before you got your period? Your pregnancy hormones are having a similar effect. Try to think past your immediate emotions. Speak with your practitioner about your mood swings and ask for advice. Depression is never to be taken lightly, but the zany emotional swings pregnancy can produce are probably not serious signs of a clinical problem. You are just beginning an intense life-altering experience and it's only normal to be fearful, dreamy, ambivalent, anxious, moody, confused, and ecstatically happy.

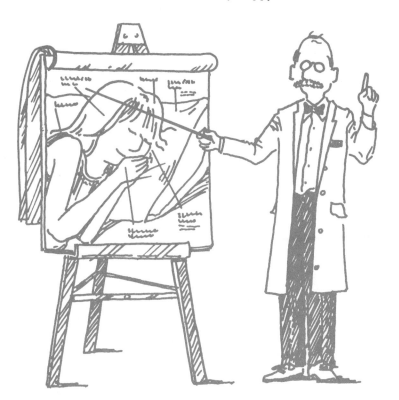

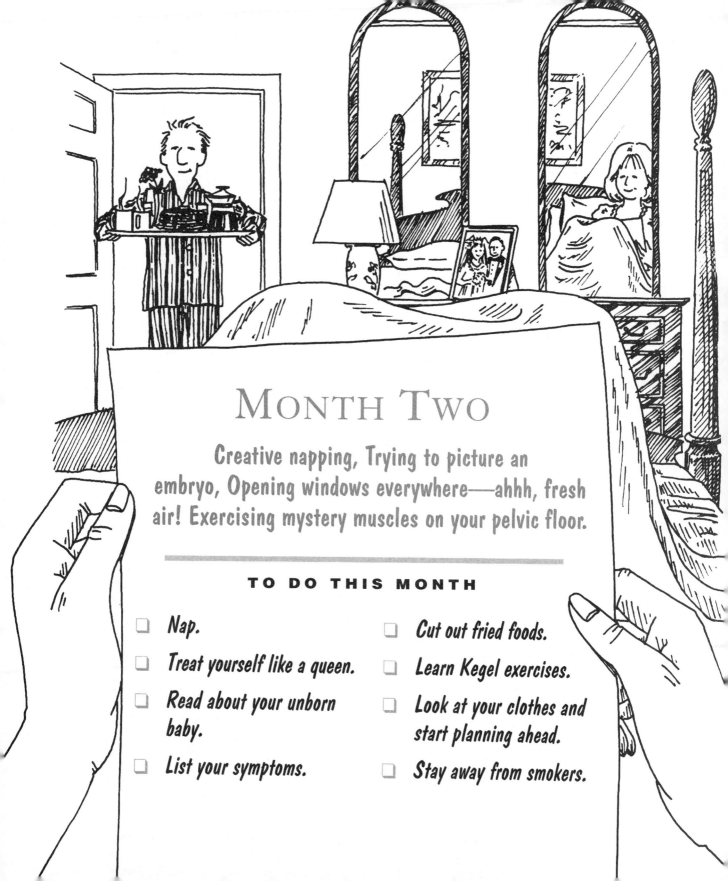

MONTH TWO

Creative napping, Trying to picture an
embryo, Opening windows everywhere—ahhh, fresh
air! Exercising mystery muscles on your pelvic floor.

TO DO THIS MONTH

- ☐ Nap.
- ☐ Treat yourself like a queen.
- ☐ Read about your unborn baby.
- ☐ List your symptoms.
- ☐ Cut out fried foods.
- ☐ Learn Kegel exercises.
- ☐ Look at your clothes and start planning ahead.
- ☐ Stay away from smokers.

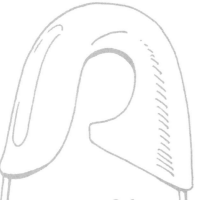

Soooo . . . Other
Pregnant Women
Have These
Symptoms, Too:

- Tender breasts
- Fatigue
- Occasional dizziness
- Frequent urination
- Nausea
- Insomnia
- Constipation
- Indigestion
- Stomach as well as intestinal gas
- Runny nose
- Headaches
- Vaginal discharge
- Cravings for strange foods; aversions to old favorites
- Weird changes in skin and hair

Welcome to the second month of your pregnancy! Can you imagine a time more filled with secret joy, hold-your-breath anxiety, and dramatic shifts away from what had been your normal, everyday existence? Where life once revolved around you and perhaps your mate, now it has become more complicated. You, in fact, are no longer yourself. You are thinking and actually living for *two*, and one of this pair has yet to be born. Slow down. Take it easy. Be kind to yourself. You can have it all and do it all, of course, but you've got to be aware of how important your own needs are. Racing through life, trying to get it all done, all finished, all ready, every day, all day long, is not the answer. You'll drive yourself nuts. *Nap* is an important three letter word for you right now.

What Are You Feeling Emotionally?

Sanford Matthews, M.D., insists that "From the very first positive news on your pregnancy test to childbirth, there is a tremendous force, a tremendous environmental drive subverting your individuality. It can be a perfectly wonderful experience—and it often is—but it can also be a perplexing time . . . a time when nothing is grounded, not even the size of your ring finger." Matthews believes that "The hormones being marshaled to protect and nurture your pregnancy affect your brain." You may experience what he calls "a chemical brainwash."

Some women choose to wait until they are well into their tenth, eleventh, or twelfth week to tell anyone other than the man in their life that they are pregnant. Most miscarriages occur in these first few weeks of pregnancy, so sometimes announcing a pregnancy too soon can make life uncomfortable later if you lose the baby. The burden of carrying such a big secret can be either deliciously pleasant or uncomfortably weighty. Some want to shout the good news from every rooftop immediately. That's fine, too. No matter which approach you choose, this second month is a time of settling into the impact of your new state.

Oh Baby . . . Inside Secrets Now

- Embedded in the side of your uterus, your embryo is about the size of a small grape, or perhaps half an inch, at the beginning of this second month of pregnancy. Its head is rather large and bent toward the chest at about week seven of development. A face is beginning to be discernible, but eyes, apparent because of a black pigment beneath the skin, are on the sides of the head and closely sealed.

- A heart has begun to circulate blood through the tiny body and signs of a nearly completed nervous system can be seen.

- In the second month of prenatal life, your baby's brain grows rapidly. The right and left hemispheres are formed and cranial nerves branch out. Membranes appear around the brain and fluid protects the tiny mass of cells. By the end of this month, this brain is working and exerting its influence on the way the unborn child moves.

- At eight weeks, the embryo can be called a *fetus*, which simply means "young one."

- Arms and legs are clearly in place but at the ends of each, the embryo has only little clefts, which will soon turn into hands, fingers, feet, and toes. Soon, these little feet will begin to kick. Muscles, which have also been forming, start exercising just as they will in the outside world.

- Not yet fully formed are the lungs, intestines, liver, and kidneys. Important internal organ systems are nearly completed by the end of this second month and your unborn baby will have grown to about an inch long. To put this size into perspective, try picturing a plump strawberry. Heart chambers form and the heartbeat becomes very human in pattern. Lungs enlarge. Bones develop. The digestive and circulatory systems keep growing. Although your fetus is not really eating anything in a digestive sense, the stomach is already secreting gastric juices. The liver is also manufacturing blood cells for bone marrow.

- A recognizable face appears with a little nose and the jaw moves into place to make way for a mouth. The tongue isn't far behind. Later in the month, eyes shift from the sides to the front of the face. Tissues from either side come together to form the face and nose and the buds of twenty baby teeth can be seen by experts.

- Inside the ears, the parts of the body responsible for hearing and equilibrium grow.

- Although you probably can't feel anything yet, your baby begins to move around inside his or her safe watery world. Don't worry. Most expectant moms don't become sensitive to these flutterings until about the eighteenth to twentieth week of pregnancy. The first fetal movements are often called *quickening*.

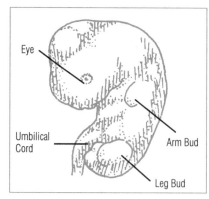

At seven weeks, the embryo is about the size of a grape, roughly one-half-inch.

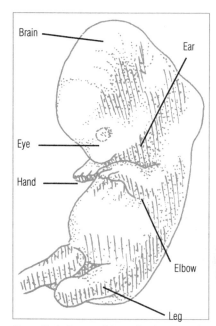

Now called a fetus at eight weeks, the arm and leg buds have already grown to distinct limbs. The fetus is one inch.

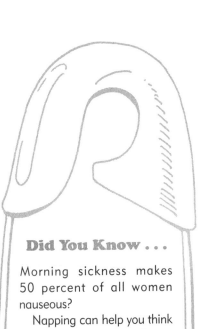

Did You Know . . .

Morning sickness makes 50 percent of all women nauseous?

Napping can help you think straight for up to ten hours after you wake up?

Not drinking enough water can make you feel sleepy?

The nicotine in cigarettes slows up the blood flow to the placenta, which is keeping your baby alive inside you?

Let's Get Physical

Even though your pregnancy may be noticeable to outsiders only until after the sixteenth week, you know you are pregnant because you just don't *feel* like your old self. You've missed two menstrual periods by now. The fetus has grown 240 times in length and a million, yes a million, times in weight. You may have some annoying symptoms straight on through the next seven months. Other aches, pains, or upsets are going to be particularly troublesome right now but will pass. Check through the following to see if you can find something that's been troubling you . . . and the answer you need.

Sick to your stomach . . . and not necessarily in the morning.

Morning sickness, which affects about 50 percent of all pregnant women, may be one of the very first signals of pregnancy. First mentioned by ancient Egyptians as long ago as 2000 B.C., your nausea is not always confined to the morning. An upset stomach and outright vomiting can happen at any particular time of day, making us all wonder why it isn't called all-day sickness. These facts may not make you feel any better, but here's the truth: triggered by the smell of certain foods, odors, or the smoke from a lit cigarette, morning sickness is usually worse for first-time moms-to-be. Studies indicate that you are also more likely to feel sick if you are under age twenty, if you weigh more than 170 pounds, if you are having twins, and if you are a nonsmoker. The extent of your morning sickness can run the gamut, from a case of mild queasiness during the first twelve weeks to severe vomiting for nine long months.

There are dramatic cases when expectant mothers vomit almost continually throughout pregnancy. A good friend of mine who gave birth to a healthy baby boy just last year, spent nine months of pure hell, throwing up so continually and so violently that she had to be hospitalized more than once for intravenous feeding to bring her symptoms under control and restore her biochemistry. Called *hyperemesis gravidarum*, this condition is reserved for only a small percentage of women.

Exactly why do you feel so sick while other pregnant women seem to bounce through the day eating everything in sight? No one

Twins? Multiples?

If twins run in your family, you certainly have an increased chance of doubling your pregnancy efforts. Yet, if you did not take fertility drugs to get pregnant, your likelihood of naturally conceived twins has actually dropped in recent years. Fertility treatments do increase the chances that you will become pregnant with more than one baby.

- You will have fraternal twins if two separate eggs are fertilized by two separate sperm. Three times more common than identical twins, and based on heredity, these fraternal fetuses have their own placentas, may even be different sexes, and may not look more like each other than ordinary brothers and sisters in the same family.

- When a single fertilized egg separates into two distinct halves, identical twins are the result. These unborn babies share the same placenta, are always the same sex, and will have the same genetic makeup and similar physical characteristics.

- Carrying two or more babies will put a lot more stress on your body and your doctor is going to monitor you much more closely than if you were expecting one baby. Early detection of the babies using ultrasounds and by taking blood tests to measure your hormone levels will help keep you on track. A multiple pregnancy means you are more likely to deliver prematurely and the aim is to keep the babies growing inside you as long as possible. Neils Lauerson, M.D., a clinical professor at New York Medical College, explains, "A one-baby pregnancy is 40 weeks long, but for a multiple birth, gestation is shorter. Twins are normally born in 37 weeks, triplets in 35 weeks, and quadruplets in 34 weeks."

- Get ready to visit your doctor's office much more often, perhaps every two to three weeks even in this first trimester. And be sure to ask about how altering your own life can help make your pregnancy go smoother. For instance, some experts believe that you may want to sit back and sit still after the fifth month. Plan ahead. Get excited and read as much as you can. There are even organizations for parents of twins or multiples. (See Appendix, pg. 288.) Join early. Learn all you can now when you are better rested than you will be after the births.

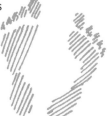

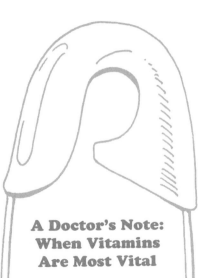

A Doctor's Note: When Vitamins Are Most Vital

While vitamins are recommended throughout pregnancy, especially folic acid, they are only really essential in the last seven to ten weeks when fetal growth is most rapid. If I have a pregnant patient who has been very ill to the point of being kept on IV fluids, and she can't handle vitamins any earlier, her baby can develop very well if she takes vitamins in those last weeks of growth.

— Howard Berk, M.D.

really knows exactly why, but there are a few credible theories. Experts like Dr. Lauerson believe that "The cause of morning sickness may likely be the level of HCG (human chorionic gonadotropin) or the pregnancy hormone in the blood. HCG rises a few days after a missed period, which is when morning sickness usually starts. Continuously secreted by the brain and the placenta, HCG peaks at about eight weeks and dramatically falls at about twelve weeks. Suddenly a woman who has been sick and vomiting for months will awaken with barely a discomfort." This twelve-week phenomenon doesn't always hold true for everyone, however. The National Institutes of Health studied 8,000 pregnant women in two separate surveys done during the 1980s and reported that not only were 29 percent nauseous up to Week 16, but 25 percent were also getting sick well into their twentieth week.

Another morning sickness theory proposed by Swedish researchers and that expounds on this HCG connection is that you are more likely to be nauseous if your fertilized ovum came from your right ovary. As odd as it may seem, here's the explanation behind this idea: You have an important ovarian vein that carries hormones from the ovary directly to your liver on the right side. The research team theorized that having your unborn baby originate on this right side brings on a kind of hormonal overload delivering an extra wallop to your liver and making you sick. In their work back in 1986, women whose eggs had been released from the left side were less likely to have nausea.

Simply knowing why you feel sick is probably of little comfort. What you need are ideas to calm your stomach. Here are ways to combat morning sickness collected from ex-pregnant women as well as pregnancy experts. Some of the ideas seem to be in direct contradiction with one another, but each has worked for some women:

Morning sickness solutions

- Try eating dry crackers, toast, or fruit. If you actually do feel sickest in the morning, keep a box of crackers by the side of your bed, and eat something as soon as you wake up.
- Eliminate fried or highly seasoned foods.

- Go with many mini-meals instead of three big square meals a day.
- Drink lots of water but not with foods. Wait at least thirty minutes before or after eating to take a drink.
- Stick with beverages that are either very hot or very cold. If liquids of any kind are treating your stomach unkindly, get your share via fruits and vegetables. Eat lettuce, for instance. It's mostly water.
- Try fruit sorbets, ice cream, yogurt, or milk shakes.
- Even when you don't feel like eating, force yourself. An empty stomach can make you even more queasy than one partially filled.
- Complex carbohydrates may go down easier than other foods. Along with crackers and toast, nibble on dry cereal, bread sticks, rice cakes, plain popcorn (skip the butter), and baked potatoes.
- Some expectant moms praise the power of proteins alone. However, hard-boiled eggs and cheese are wiser choices than red meat.
- Steer clear of smells that can trigger occasions of nausea if you can. For instance, if the scent of freshly brewing coffee sets your stomach rolling, ask your mate to pick up his morning brew outside your vicinity. When you have to cook, open the kitchen windows or turn on an exhaust fan.
- Prenatal vitamins, which contain iron, can irritate your digestive tract. If you are experiencing serious bouts of morning sickness, speak with your doctor about altering your vitamin or even taking a vacation from your vitamin regimen.
- The B vitamins taken as supplements, as well as foods rich in them can help, according to Dr. Lauerson. Check with your own doctor, but consider taking a B complex and B_6.
- Move slowly. Aim for tranquillity. Sit on the side of your bed for a few minutes each morning. Let your stomach settle before you attempt any quick moves.
- Ask your doctor about medications especially if you are so sick that you are worried about your unborn baby. New, anti-emetic drugs can be used with marked success under

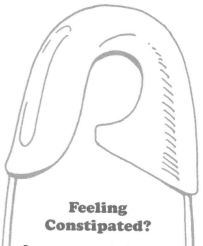

Feeling Constipated?

Progesterone, one of the hormones now circulating wildly in your system, relaxes the gastrointestinal muscles in the walls of your intestines and slows down bowel movements. If you are constipated, you are not alone. More than half of all expectant mothers suffer from constipation at some point during their pregnancies.

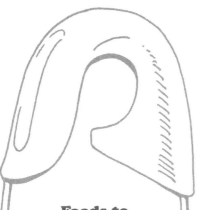

Foods to Reconsider Right Now

Here are some gas-producing foods to watch and cut down—at least until your stomach settles:

- Apples
- Bananas
- Beans
- Broccoli
- Cabbage
- Cauliflower
- Corn
- Cucumbers
- Meringues
- Milk
- Oats and other high-fiber grains
- Onions
- Turnips

the care of a doctor. Emetrol, a mint-flavored liquid, is available in pharmacies over-the-counter. Maalox and other antacids may be able to relieve symptoms, too. Antihistamines have also been known to quiet queasy stomachs. However, do *not* take anything without the backing of your doctor. Always ask first.

How to get going . . .

- Avoid taking laxatives if you can, unless they are prescribed by your doctor. Look around for natural remedies, instead. For instance, drinking lots of water. Can you stomach up to ten or twelve eight-ounce glasses a day? If so, this increase in fluids should make your gastrointestinal tract feel better.
- Try eating fiber-rich foods, such as prunes, figs, whole fruits and vegetables, including the skins or peels, seeds, and whole-grain breads or cereals with bran. They work as natural laxatives. Fruit juices also help.
- Stay active. If you've stopped or slowed up your exercise routine because you are pregnant, this lack of movement could be aggravating your constipation problem. Go for a twenty-minute walk at least once a day.

If constipation has become such a nightmare for you that you are developing hemorrhoids, speak with your doctor. (Go to Month Four for more about hemorrhoids.)

You've got the gassy, bloated blues.

Guess what? Sometimes you just can't win. If you've been eating lots of fiber-rich foods in your quest to end constipation, you could end up with good old gas. Stomach rumbling, burping, a feeling of fullness, and the overwhelming urge to pass gas in the most embarrassing situations are just a few of the symptoms pregnant women have to endure.

- Gas-X is perfectly safe and can make you feel better.

Worried About Wetting Your Underpants? Try These Two Exercises

Okay, even if you are still exercising regularly, still walking several times a week, still taking your aerobic dance classes, or still lifting those weights . . . you need to add new exercises to your daily routine now that you are pregnant. To improve bladder control now in your first trimester, you should start pelvic floor exercises. These routines will also be great for labor, delivery, and for helping you recover faster after the baby is born.

The hammock of muscles that support your bowel, bladder, and womb on the floor of your pelvis needs to stay strong and elastic. When you are pregnant, these muscles get softer and spongier. When you add this to the weight of your growing baby directly above, you can end up with a problem. You feel heavy and uncomfortable. When you sneeze, laugh, or cough suddenly, you may even end up leaking a bit of urine.

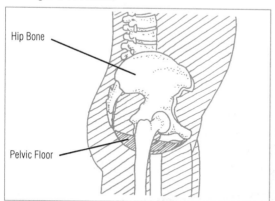

The pelvic floor forms as part of the pelvis and serves to cradle the baby in the womb. Kegel exercises help to strengthen this area.

You can do pelvic floor exercises anytime, anywhere, and will soon want to do them up to one hundred times a day, but not all at once. Known as *Kegel exercises*, they can be done at your convenience and no one even really needs to know you are exercising. Do them while watching television, riding in a car, combing your hair, or before climbing out of bed in the morning.

1. With your legs slightly apart, tighten and release the muscles around your vagina. There are two techniques to help you figure out how to do this. First, put your hand over your pubic bones and contract your vaginal muscles as far up to your fingers. Do this five, ten, twenty times. Work your way up to one hundred a day.

The next time you are going to the bathroom, stop the flow of urine right in the middle. Then start again. Then stop again. Those are the muscles you want to strengthen. Howard Shapiro, M.D., a Connecticut obstetrician-gynecologist, tells mothers-to-be to "tighten the muscles of the buttocks as though trying to prevent the escape of feces. This same group of muscles is used to stop the flow of urine." Dr. Shapiro believes, "If you perform these exercises diligently, you will note improvement in your ability to tighten the muscles surrounding the vagina and perineum (pelvic floor)."

2. Tighten and release your vaginal muscles, but take a slower approach. In fact, as you tighten, count to six. As you release, count to four. Tighten to six. Relax to four. Breathe normally and resist that temptation to hold your breath.

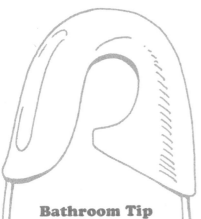

- Stick to small meals because they won't overload your digestive tract.
- Don't gulp. Gulping down anything, especially carbonated drinks, can also add to your angst.
- Take yoga. Anxiety alone can work your body up to a frenzy. Don't forget to tell the instructor that you are pregnant.
- Check with your doctor and discuss your diet.

Bathroom Tip

Empty your bladder completely every time you go to the bathroom. Think you are finished? Sit still for a second. Try to go again.

You need to urinate frequently all day and sometimes all night long.

You might have a urinary tract infection, which can lead to premature labor, so speak with your doctor about your symptoms. However, early in pregnancy, frequent urination can be caused by progesterone relaxing the muscles in your bladder. The nerves that direct the need to go to the bathroom are also sending signals to your brain even though you may have just recently urinated. In your second trimester, this overwhelming need to race to the nearest bathroom should ease up. Later the problem may return when the fetus drops down into your pelvis and puts pressure on your kidneys. If nightly trips out of bed are ruining your sleep, drink less in the evenings.

You are utterly exhausted.

Fatigue is caused by your hormones, especially progesterone, which seems to be the culprit for quite a few of these meddlesome side effects of pregnancy. Even when researchers inject this hormone into laboratory animals in experiments, the subjects become extremely sleepy. Give in to the feeling if you can. Rest as much as you can. In the next trimester, you probably won't be as washed out. In these days of rush-rush, hurry-hurry, it's hard to give in to the urge to nap and to keep in mind that you are giving your unborn baby a peaceful growing environment. Physicians believe that extreme tiredness is a way of forcing you to rest.

More ways your body says . . . "Yes, you're pregnant!"

Subtle and not-so-subtle physical changes can make you fearful, unless you anticipate them as predictable and quite normal. Here are more ways your body may be saying, "Something's happening!" this month.

- Your vagina feels full, congested, and actually bigger than it used to be. You may also have more secretions. An increase in the amount of clear or white mucus is normal unless you are sore. If that happens, let your doctor know right away because you may have developed an infection. Report any itching, pain, or colored or foul-smelling discharge.

- Your breasts are growing and not just in size. The areolas, the pigmented areas around the nipple, have changed. They are getting bigger and are darker in color. Veins in your breast are more noticeable and could be painful, sensitive, or actually throbbing, especially when in contact with a tight bra or any pressure.

- Your need for oxygen increases. I used to drive my husband crazy with my craving for fresh air, no matter what season of the year. Even in winter, I simply had to leave the window wide open at night for that night air.

- You may also feel faint or dizzy on occasion because your blood pressure is lower than it used to be. Several cardiovascular changes are taking place. By the time you finish this first trimester, your heart will be pumping up to 50 percent more blood than before, the walls of your blood vessels will be looser, and the total volume of plasma will be up. Fainting can also be caused by low blood sugar or not enough iron.

- Your gums may bleed because the tissues of your mouth are softer. If they become inflamed, speak with your dentist. Schedule a thorough cleaning for your teeth right away and don't forget to floss.

Yikes . . . What Are You Going to Wear?

Even though you probably haven't outgrown the waistlines on your skirts, slacks, and dresses yet, maternity clothes are beckoning. What will you need? Where will you shop? Have maternity clothes changed from your mother's day? How do other women get through this?

"You've got to try hard not to feel dumpy or let yourself look like a slob even if you aren't reporting to a job during your pregnancy."

—J. S., A FORMER SYSTEMS ANALYST
PREGNANT FOR THE SECOND TIME

"This is my first pregnancy and I'm dressing to please myself as much as for anyone else. It's so important for my self-esteem."

—S. S., PSYCHOTHERAPIST WHO WENT
BACK TO SCHOOL FOR A BUSINESS DEGREE

"Near the end of my first trimester, I would get up in the morning and end up trying on ten different outfits before I found one that snapped, buttoned or didn't fit skintight."

—S. D., A NURSE

"When my mother was pregnant, she wore a lot of black. She tells me that she was happy to have become pregnant in the late fifties because that was the turning point for dowdy to delightful. The elastic panel was in, drawstring tops had arrived, and she was able to bypass the potato sacks they had been trying to pass off on pregnant women."

—M. F., A FORMER FASHION BUYER'S ASSISTANT

"Even though something might look ridiculous on a hanger, try it on. This is the one stage of your life when you can't trust those old clothing instincts you thought you had narrowed down. Seriously, I never believed that an extra long sweater with matching leg warmers would look anything but ridiculous on a pregnant me. Yet, believe me, I wore it and received compliments."

—B. V., FULL-TIME MOM

The Fine Art of Napping

Although napping is never going to be a substitute for a good night's sleep, a nap a day can help you think straight for up to ten hours afterward. Another napping benefit: Some experts believe that thirty minutes of snoozing can lower your chance of heart disease.

Nap-Taking Tips:

- Can't carve out hours of free time? Steal five, ten, or just fifteen minutes from the rest of your busy day and close your eyes. A short sleep will still benefit you and your unborn baby.
- Don't choose a chair. Find a bed or stretch out on the couch.
- Don't sleep stuffed (after a big meal) or starved (with a stomach growling for food).
- Set the room temperature for the mid-sixties. If you are too hot or too cold, you won't be able to drift off.
- Watch your caffeine consumption.
- Save problems for when you wake up. Let go of anxieties. You can find the answers later.
- Develop a nap ritual. One woman I know, who worked full time in an office until the day before her baby was born, took an exercise mat to work so she could roll it out in the afternoon and close her eyes. If you have an office door to close out the world, do so. If that's not possible and you can't even find space to stretch out, settle for a catnap. Just close your eyes and rest.

For Your Information:

- Most people start to slump after twelve hours of being awake. You can blame sleepiness on being pregnant, of course, but if you are trying to push yourself through a long day of unending activity, you can also blame it on your body rhythms.
- Drink water when you feel fatigued. Your brain is 75 percent water, and every chemical reaction that occurs in your body uses water. If you are dehydrated, you will be less productive.
- Don't slouch. Good posture—neck lengthened, chin in, shoulders back, head up—can actually give you 30 percent more lung capacity.
- Stay away from sweets. Sugars offer an instant pick-up, but your body will droop as soon as the extra insulin is churned out.

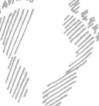

Thank goodness you aren't pregnant for the seventh time in seven years in pre–Revolutionary War America. If that were true, out would come your corset with its uncomfortable stays designed to choke back your growing belly. There was no such thing as a maternity dress or, certainly not, a pair of comfortable jeans. You would be wearing your regular dresses as long as you could and when you could not squeeze your body into a single one, you just didn't see the light of day until after your delivery. That's called *confinement*, which is exactly how pregnant women spent the better part of their pregnancies. Not only was it unattractive but one expert in the maternity fashion industry insists that it was also "inefficient, uncomfortable, and unhealthy. Women referred to it privately in their diaries and letters as "the dreaded apparition" and "the greatest of earthly miseries."

The first maternity dress—a cheap, cotton wrap-around house dress—was mass manufactured in the early 1900s. Yet, it wasn't until the 1930s that anyone thought of making clothes for making pregnant pretty. My great aunt Frances had three daughters and a son seventy-some years ago. "We would wear our cotton house dresses until they began to pull at the seams," she once told me. Then, you had to have a dressmaker (or if you could sew yourself, of course, you would do it) cut the side seams of your dresses from the armholes to the hemline and insert long triangular panels of matching material called gussets. By placing one point of the triangle under the arm-hole, and then letting the rest of the insert extend all the way to the original hem of your dress, you could end up with a voluminous dress to take you through your pregnancy. If you could stand wearing that same dress after the birth, it was no big deal to remove the gussets from the dress and reattach the original seams.

Edna and Elsie's Great Idea

Along with a slew of tradespeople who stepped in to sell women maternity clothes back in the 1930s were two sisters from University Park, Texas. In 1937, Edna and Elsie couldn't believe how terrible Edna looked when she was expecting her first child. Recalls Edna, "Elsie insisted that she was going to make me something to wear that would hang evenly. And the only thing we could both think of to do the trick was to cut a hole in the stomach portion of

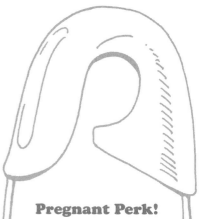

the skirt, and then cover it with a long tunic top." Neither sister understood why Edna should have to sacrifice her sense of style and simply "get through the pregnancy" and back to her own clothes. The outfit they created was black and rather sophisticated for the time. It also launched the sisters into the maternity clothes design business.

What You Will Need to Get Dressed

Oftentimes, maternity wardrobe recommendations are based on two-season thinking. You are told that you fall into either spring–summer or autumn–winter. Well, anyone who has ever been pregnant will intimately understand the fallacy of such thinking. If you are due in October, you can't buy clothes with a fall mentality. What about those hot July and August days of summer when you are very much pregnant? An October due date puts you right in the middle of three seasons, especially if you live in a Northern or Middle-Atlantic state where weather patterns run the gamut. Even if you live in Southern California or the southernmost tip of Florida, it may be helpful to know what lies ahead when it comes to getting dressed in the morning.

Before You Go Clothes Shopping

Here are basic ideas for what you may need to have in your closet in the months to come. Start with the essentials, such as underwear, night clothes, T-shirts, exercise wear, or perhaps a pair of black leggings for pulling on beneath big shirts and sweaters. Some women are truly gifted at getting by with less. Others absolutely need more variation and changes in order to feel happy and comfortable. With today's assortment of stretch fabrics that actually let your skin breathe too, you may be able to get by far longer with your own clothes, completely avoiding the maternity clothes issue or at least delaying it until that last trimester. Or, you could start borrowing basics from your husband's side of the closet. Man-tailored shirts, suit vests, his baggy sweaters, elastic waist jogging shorts, his large T-shirts, windbreakers, barn jackets, and outerwear can help you stretch your clothing dollars.

Pregnant Perk!

Everyone needs a quiet hour, half-hour, or even ten minutes of serenity a day. Highly successful people claim that it sharpens their minds and relaxes their bodies. When you are pregnant, you especially need to sit quietly and daydream a little each day. If utter stillness makes you antsy to get up and move, try browsing in a bookstore, walking around the block, or pursuing any kind of mindless, yet pleasurable, activity.

Your lifestyle will also dictate what kind of clothes you need. If you are a lawyer working full time and expected to appear in court, then you'll be thinking suits. However, if you are a full-time at-home mother, you'll be interested in more casual clothes. A friend who has recently been pregnant can also allow you borrowing opportunities.

If You Are Due in January or February
You will outgrow your waistband by August–September.
You'll need:

- Dresses

    1 casual. If you are being careful with money, consider a jumper that can be dressed up or down and in a color that won't be out of place in either early September or all the way into February. Be creative. Look for something unusual but basic. How about khaki?

    1 dressy. If you choose a seasonless fabric, you'll be able to wear this early in September and into those colder months. Something with three-quarter length sleeves could also be versatile . . . not too long to be out of place in warm weather or too short to look bare when it gets colder.

- Pants

    1 pair of jeans

    2 pairs of corduroys or gabardine. If you make one pair black, you can dress them up for an evening in December; and coordinated with a black sweater, you can throw it on and feel pulled together.

    1 pair of wool or gabardine, trouser-leg, dressy slacks.

- Tops

    3 sweaters

    4 shirts or pullovers (Think ahead to the holiday season for one of them.)

- Miscellaneous

    1 sweatsuit. If you are pregnant over the Christmas and New Year's holidays, there may be a lot of pressure to be ready to dress up. So don't spend your entire budget early in the fall.

If You Are Due in March or April

You will outgrow your waistband by October–November.
You'll need:

- Dresses

   2 casual. The selection in maternity dresses is often bigger and better than separates, and because you can afford to concentrate on winter, look for two dresses that can get you through a day at work or at home and right on into a casual evening.

   1 dressy (The holidays will definitely be upon you.)

- Pants

   1 pair of jeans

   2 pairs of winter-weight (Corduroy is fine, but perhaps velvet might work because this fabric stretches so decently and has become so much more versatile in recent years.)

   1 pair of good wool or gabardine slacks

- Tops

   3 sweaters (They may take a beating in terms of stretching and tugging.)

   4 long-sleeved tops (Blouses, knits, winter pullover, or T-shirt style.)

- Miscellaneous

   You will need an exclusively winter wardrobe, so a denim jumper might be a good option. Look for a style that suits your shape best. Try on as many styles as you can find. Some have bigger armholes than others.

If You Are Due in May or June

You will outgrow your waistband by December–January.
You'll need:

- Dresses

   1 casual. Think spring, even though you may be shopping in February or March. You'll want this casual number to take you into June, if possible.

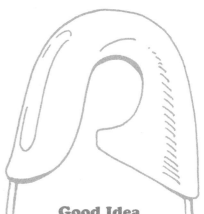

Good Idea

If you happen to be married to a large-sized guy who has a tuxedo he doesn't wear anymore, these slacks, when worn with suspenders, are often great for dressing up or down. Even if you don't have the luxury of home-grown tuxedo pants, you may be able to find a pair at a thrift shop.

1 dressy. Make this a simple style so you can wear it for lunch or dress it up for dinner.

1 sundress. If it is a solid color, you may be able to wear it with a blouse or T-shirt in the cooler months and then all by itself when the weather changes in June.

- Pants

    1 pair of jeans

    1 pair of corduroys. Pick a pale color so it won't seem out of place in May. The weight will be right for March, too.

    1 pair of cotton trousers. Make these dark-colored slacks so they will work early in your pregnancy and then again with a summer top toward the end. For instance, black cotton pants can be sweater-layered early on and then used again with a summer top in May or June.

    1 pair of good shorts. In addition to simple running shorts, you'll want something that won't look out of place when you go for a walk on a sweltering day in June.

- Tops

    2 sweaters. Think about buying one wool or a wool blend and one cotton for warmer weather.

    3 shirts. If you choose a long-sleeved version when you are buying in March or April, why not get something that can be rolled up for a lighter look? A style that is tight at your wrists won't roll up far enough.

    2 T-shirt tops for early summer and late spring. Buy carefully and you may be able to layer these purchases, for earlier wear.

- Miscellaneous

    1 jumper

If You Are Due in July or August

You will outgrow your waistband by February–March. You'll need:

- Dresses

    1 casual

    1 dressy

    1 sundress

- Pants

    3 pairs of cotton trousers. You may not need jeans if you can squeeze into your regular jeans until early spring.
    1 pair of shorts

- Tops

    2 sweaters. Pick a blend and a color that will span the seasons and one that can definitely be worn by itself or with a shirt.
    1 long-sleeved maternity top
    2 summer shirts or T-shirts

- Miscellaneous

    1 bathing suit

If You Are Due in September or October

You will outgrow your waistband by April–May. You'll need:

- Dresses

    1 dressy
    2 sundresses. Make sure that one can be worn as a jumper with a blouse or T-shirt underneath.

- Pants

    2 pairs of cotton trousers. By choosing a dark color for one, you can help it stretch through three seasons.
    2 pairs of shorts, 1 casual, 1 dressy

- Tops

    1 summer-to-fall sweater
    3 summer tops chosen with layering in mind
    1 long-sleeved maternity top

- Miscellaneous

    1 seersucker jumper or jumpsuit
    1 bathing suit

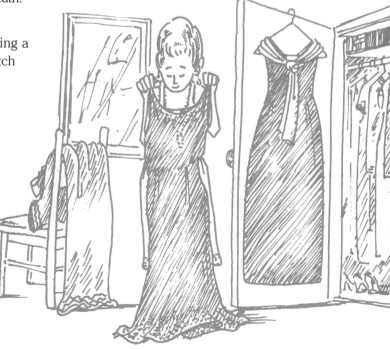

If You Are Due in November or December
You will outgrow your waistband by June–July. You'll need:

- Dresses
    1 casual
    1 dressy (The holiday season will arrive when you are at your biggest.)
    1 sundress

- Pants
    1 pair of jeans
    1 pair of corduroy or lightweight wool or gabardine slacks. Look for something in a light corduroy so you can wear them into early October with a sweater.
    1 pair of cotton trousers

- Tops
    2 sweaters, one lightweight and one woolly for a winter's day
    2 long-sleeved shirts
    2 short summer tops

- Miscellaneous
    1 bathing suit

More Tips for Looking Great Later This Year

- *What size should you buy?* Most women wear their regular size in dresses and tops. However, if you are busty, you may want to go up. Because most maternity clothes are cut larger and looser, you can probably check adjacent sizes for all your needs. One size smaller or larger doesn't make any difference. In slacks or skirts, you will probably be one or two sizes larger than your normal number. Most women gain weight in their thighs and this is where you need that extra room. Though some manufacturers claim that women should always buy their regular size, this isn't always true. I've seen friends who have become upset when they couldn't squeeze into a size four or six pair of slacks. Aim for the rack near your old size and be creative.

- *Why should you spend money on clothes that will fit you for only six months?* Because you have fewer choices in your closet, you'll probably be wearing these maternity items much more frequently than your non-maternity clothes. You will get your money's worth. Maternity clothes are worn three times more often during a busy seven-month period of your life and many women rely on them after the baby arrives, too. With so much else happening to throw you off balance emotionally, it will make you feel better about yourself if you make the effort to look good as your body changes.

- *How can you tell if the dress you try on in the first trimester is actually going to fit seven months later?* Check to see if the shoulder seams are in their proper places. Then, grab some of the fabric right at your bust line to see if it will give another inch or two. If it will, the stomach area will undoubtedly stretch as well.

- *Why can't you wear large-size regular clothes?* You can. Sometimes, this tactic works just perfectly. Be careful about hemlines, however. The front of the dress, for instance, will sneak up and the back will dip down later in pregnancy. Sometimes an outfit is worth buying if you think it can be altered or you know you will wear it for part of your pregnancy and then again after the baby comes.

- *Will I need special tops if I am going to breast-feed my baby?* Not necessarily. Some of your maternity tops are definitely going to have to merge with your postpartum wardrobe. Keep in mind that unbuttoning a blouse with one hand while cradling a baby with the other makes it pretty impossible to appear modest at the same time. Though some experts suggest button-front shirts for breast-feeding moms, soft turtlenecks and loose-fitting T-shirts that can be pulled up may be more useful. Buttoned shirts are best when you need to see exactly what you are doing, if you are in bed nursing your baby, or if you aren't skilled in hooking or unhooking the nursing bra. Pull-up tops are certainly more private, however.

Should You Take Prenatal Vitamins?

While some experts question whether you need to supplement a nutritionally well-balanced diet with a daily vitamin and mineral tablet, most practitioners feel that every pregnant woman can benefit. You certainly don't want to risk a deficiency in anything while your fetus is growing and you definitely need extra folic acid and perhaps additional iron, so prenatal vitamins may be just what your body and your baby need. Dosages are not excessive or dangerous. Different brands contain varying concentrations of vitamins and minerals, so if one particular manufacturer's blend upsets your system, try another. Some even have stool softeners to counteract the problem of constipation, a common side effect of iron supplementation. On the labels, expect to see Vitamin A, D, E, C, Folic Acid, B_1, B_2, Niacinamide, B_6, B_{12}, Calcium, Iodine, Magnesium, Copper, Zinc, Biotin, and Pantothenic Acid.

I Was Wondering . . .

Will the bottle of champagne I shared with my husband on the night we conceived our baby be harmful? I've been worried since I suspected I was pregnant a few weeks and calculated back that this was the very night we had been celebrating our wedding anniversary. I really did overdo it that night, although usually I'm pretty careful about sticking to a glass of wine.

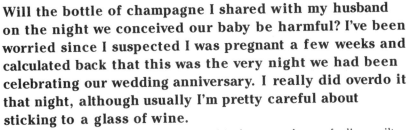

Put this night of celebration behind you and stop feeling guilty. Guilt is a waste of your time now. Binge drinking or regular abuse of alcohol when you are pregnant can cause birth defects, but an isolated episode of too much champagne probably has not harmed your unborn baby. Alcohol consumption during the first trimester is particularly troublesome, however. Niels Lauerson, M.D., a New York obstetrician and gynecologist, has stated, "In the first three months of pregnancy, when biological systems—especially the nervous system—are forming and the fetus is most vulnerable, alcohol can have a particularly damaging effect. . . .

Please note that Dr. Lauerson is discussing women who were drunk on a consistent or daily basis. Two to four drinks a week will not produce alcohol syndrome, according to Dr. Howard Berk. Lauerson believes that if you do feel the need to have a social drink, the second and third trimesters are a less worrisome time to indulge. Alcohol, he explains, absorbs your body's nutrients so "make sure you increase your intake of essential nutrients and vitamins." Unfortunately, Lauerson reports, "The FDA is unable to set a 'safe' level for alcoholic consumption during pregnancy."

Because knowledge is power, you might want to have these additional facts on hand regarding alcohol abuse during pregnancy, especially if you consider yourself a regular drinker. The information is based on a report prepared by Ashley Wivel, a medical student at Yale University School of Medicine, and appears in a wonderful Internet site, *Caring/Hygeia*, an Online Journal for Pregnancy and Neonatal Loss (http://hygeia.org). According to Wivel, one in every three hundred babies is born with some sign of what is known as fetal alcohol syndrome (FAS) because their mothers drank on a regular basis during pregnancy. Heavy drinking, including binges or daily use, is especially associated with congenital defects. Babies born with FAS show retarded growth, have central nervous system problems, and certain characteristic facial features, including a small head, a thin upper lip, a short upturned nose, a flattened nasal bridge and a general underdeveloped look of the face. Because of the critical nervous system involvement, many show tremulousness, can't suck, are hyperactive, have abnormal muscle tone, and are later diagnosed with attention deficit disorder as well as mental retardation.

Relying on alcohol out of habit or cravings can also end your pregnancy abruptly. Heavy to moderate drinkers seem to experience a higher incidence of miscarriage in the second trimester, as well as problems with the placenta. Other complications linked to alcohol use are congenital heart defects, brain abnormalities, spinal and limb defects, and urinary and genital problems.

I don't smoke but my husband does, and I'm worried about the effect of this second-hand smoke on my unborn baby. Is this a problem that should concern me?

Even though you may not be lighting up yourself, you are a passive smoker when you are with your husband and unavoidably inhaling the stream from his lit cigarette. Smoking, as well as ambient or second-hand smoking leads you to create excess carbon monoxide, which combines with hemoglobin and takes oxygen from your fetus. Smoke can lead to ear, nose, and throat infections later, as well as bronchitis, asthma, and respiratory problems. A condition known as *placental abruption*, in which the placenta actually detaches from the side of the uterus, is also related to tobacco abuse. Your risk of miscarriage increases. Ask your mate to step outside if he insists on smoking and make sure other friends and relatives do the same.

I guess you could call me an exercise nut. Are there any sports that are clearly off-limits now that I am two months pregnant?

Exercising moderately throughout your pregnancy, especially in the first trimester, is going to make you feel great and remain strong. Moderate should be your mantra, however. You are also right to be fearful of certain activities. Howard Shapiro, M.D., a Connecticut obstetrician-gynecologist and author, says that the best exercises are those that are aerobic, or done with oxygen. You can use your whole body in a continuously rhythmic motion when you are aerobically active. Walking, cycling, swimming, and cross-country skiing may make you feel great. Swimming and cycling are less weight-dependent and will be better for your growing body in that last trimester. Limit your sessions to thirty minutes. If you have been a regular ice skater, roller-blader, or roller skater, then you may need to rethink your options. First trimester activities aren't as tricky. In the third trimester, however, the extra weight can throw your balance off and make falling a problem. Your ligaments actually relax when you are expecting, so knee, ankle, and foot injuries are more likely. Although bowling, volleyball, and softball don't offer as much aerobic benefit, you can play safely when pregnant, according to Shapiro. The continuous jumping in volleyball is not great for your joints and ligaments, however. Golf, too, is an activity that should stay on your list of things to do, even though you shouldn't "expect to improve your golf swing" after the fifth month, when you have to compensate for "an increasing abdominal enlargement." Be wary of any high-impact sports. If you've been playing tennis, for instance, you might want to avoid competitive singles games and switch to doubles.

Long-distance and marathon running to the point of hyperthermia, or elevated body temperature, could be dangerous. Such strenuous exercise in the first trimester has been associated with birth defects, and later in pregnancy the stress shifts your blood away from your uterus to your legs, possibly decreasing the oxygen being carried to your unborn baby. No race is worth the danger. Other sports to put on hold are water skiing, scuba diving, horseback riding, basketball, gymnastics, field hockey, jumping rope, and softball. "If you play indoor handball, paddleball, or racquetball during the first trimester, be aware of the fact that these courts are rarely well-ventilated and pose a threat of hyperthermia," Shapiro explains. When you raise your body's temperature for a prolonged time, especially during the third, fourth, and fifth weeks of pregnancy, experts suspect that you can cause damage to the developing fetus's brain, skull, and spinal cord. Simply having a high fever because you are ill doesn't appear to be as damaging as raising your body temperature during a long physical workout. If you have been a marathon runner, you might want to know that your core body temperature can actually rise an average of 34.7 degrees Fahrenheit during a long race, according to Shapiro. However, he explains, "If a woman is aerobically fit prior to pregnancy and exercises prudently under climate-controlled conditions, hyperthermia during pregnancy can be avoided."

Before, During, and After: Exercise

Before you begin any new exercise program or aerobic dancing class, hire a personal trainer, or follow your good friends onto the tennis court, check with your practitioner. Even if the sessions are designed for expectant or postpartum moms, you should still run the idea by your practitioner first. However, even if you have never picked up a weight in your life or purchased a pair of walking shoes, pregnancy may be the perfect time to become more conscious of just what your body is capable of doing. It makes sense. It's a natural point in life to be body-focused. You'll have more energy after you move than if you opt to feel sick and stay on the couch. Honestly, a body at rest—even one feeling nauseous, weary, anxious, or enervated—is going to want to stay at rest. Yet, a body in motion—and trying to fight morning sickness, fatigue, fears, and lack of energy—is going to stay in motion and feel better in the long run.

Research conducted by Jennifer Lovejoy, a physiological psychologist at the Women's Health Research Program at the Pennington Biomedical Research Center at Louisiana State University, found that many women who find themselves out of shape and overweight later in life blame pregnancy for the turning point in their metabolism. Sure, there are good reasons to blame this life-changing event. Great

Doctor's Note: Exercise? No Sweat.

Exercise during pregnancy is still a new and somewhat controversial subject. In reality, any exercises that you have been doing all along in your life are going to be fine during pregnancy. My daughter-in-law is a triathlete who competes in these three-part athletic events, which include swimming, running, and biking the equivalent of three marathons in a row. The first time she was pregnant, she raced in a triathlon at twenty weeks. In her second pregnancy, she ran a minimum of seven miles a day. Yet, if you have never been a triathlete, you shouldn't start when you are pregnant. Only really penetrating blows will hurt the uterus.

—Howard Berk, M.D.

reasons, in fact. Having good reasons is not going to make you happy when you are still trying to squeeze into your old clothes nine months after the baby is born.

A variety of factors pile on during these crucial ten to twelve months: hormonal changes, new eating habits, stress, and no time or energy for exercise. Yet, pregnancy does not have to leave you with a legacy of twenty extra pounds. Lovejoy found that psychological factors played a key part in taking your body through a year of wild transformation. The secret may be exercise. By making exercise as much of a part of your routine as brushing your teeth or combing your hair, you stand a better chance of staying in touch with your body through all the ups, downs, ins, and outs. Think fit. Don't worry about thin. Consider yourself voluptuous, but keep on moving. Walk. Move. Take a few minutes a day to stretch and bend. You deserve it.

Clothes to Make You Move?

Yes. Find something to wear that won't make you want to cringe in front of the mirror, classmates, or your family members. Gear to get you going is more important than you might think because when you are feeling sluggish, you'll use any excuse not to move your body. Not having comfortable clothes can become a big hurdle. A comfortable, supportive bra is especially important. Nonrestrictive clothes will also let your body air out and breathe when you warm up. You don't have to think in terms of high fashion. Cotton sweats, shorts, your husband's T-shirts, a leotard in a larger size than you might ordinarily wear will all do just fine. Finding and sticking to an exercise routine can help you overcome many of the common problems of pregnancy: backaches, loss of urinary control, hemorrhoids, discomfort during sex, poor posture, muscle stiffness, and lack of energy. Activity will increase your flexibility and make it easier for you to adjust your balance through all the phases and stages of pregnancy.

Good Ideas Regarding Exercise

Stop moving

- Before you become utterly exhausted.
- If you feel pain.
- If you are short of breath.

Don't ever

- Exercise without drinking water before, during, and afterward.
- Jump up suddenly.
- Try an exercise movement that requires you to lie flat on your back after you are twenty weeks' pregnant.
- Dive into a routine without warming up with some slow steady movements first.

Warm-Up Exercises

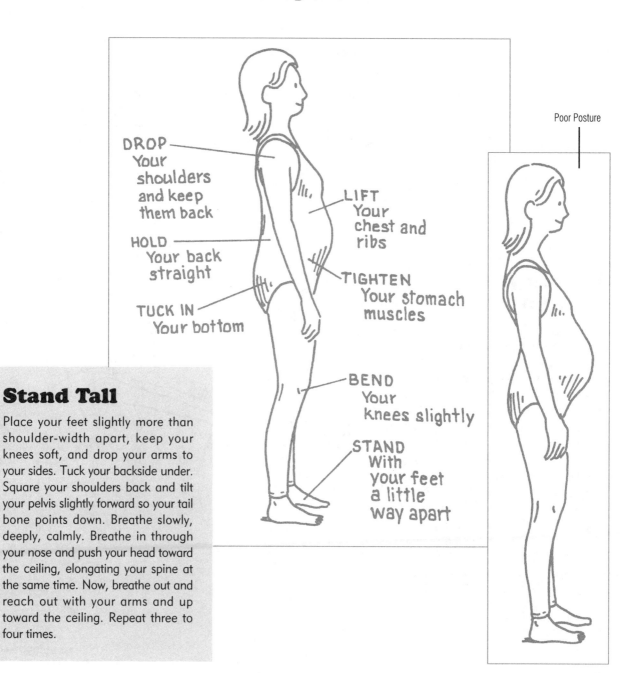

DROP
Your shoulders and keep them back

LIFT
Your chest and ribs

HOLD
Your back straight

TIGHTEN
Your stomach muscles

TUCK IN
Your bottom

BEND
Your knees slightly

STAND
With your feet a little way apart

Poor Posture

Stand Tall

Place your feet slightly more than shoulder-width apart, keep your knees soft, and drop your arms to your sides. Tuck your backside under. Square your shoulders back and tilt your pelvis slightly forward so your tail bone points down. Breathe slowly, deeply, calmly. Breathe in through your nose and push your head toward the ceiling, elongating your spine at the same time. Now, breathe out and reach out with your arms and up toward the ceiling. Repeat three to four times.

Wake Up Your Upper Body

Swing

Start this one with your arms limp and relaxed at your sides. Breathe in and out slowly. Now, swing your arms in, crossing them in front and then out to shoulder level. Repeat three to four times.

Make Circles

Increase the muscle tension in your arms a little. Keeping your elbows soft and your hands relaxed, circle your arms in toward the midpoint of your body, crossing them in front and then going up and out as if you were drawing large circles with your arms going in an inward direction. Repeat three times. Now reverse the direction and make three large circles in an outward direction.

Note: These swings and circles should make your arms and upper body feel energized.

Stretch Your Upper Back

Still standing, keep your feet slightly more than shoulder-width apart, your weight as evenly distributed as possible given your stage of pregnancy, your knees soft, and your arms at your sides. Lift your arms out to the sides to approximately shoulder level, inhaling as you lift. Exhale and slowly bring your extended arms forward at chest level, leaning slightly forward as you do and letting your pelvis tilt in just a bit. You should feel the stretch through your upper and middle back. Now, return your arms to your sides at shoulder level and contract the back muscles between your shoulder blades as you do. Exhale and repeat this stretch three or four times.

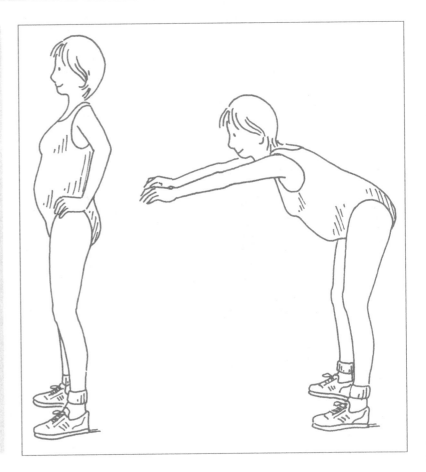

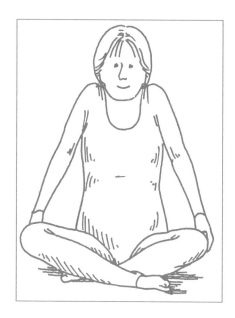

Roll Your Shoulders

Try to breathe naturally through this movement. You may be shocked by how much tension you discover in your shoulder and neck. Bring your shoulders up toward your ears and then backward in a fluid, rolling motion. Try to visualize drawing circles with your shoulders. Repeat three times. Now, reverse the movement, bringing your shoulders up and then forward. Repeat three times.

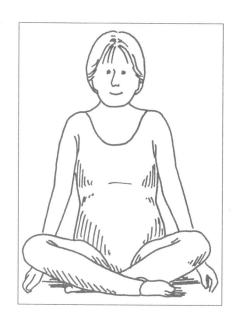

Stretch Like a Cat

Before you get tired of being on your feet, try this standing-up cat stretch to stretch and strengthen your lower back. Lower your body into a semi-sitting position with your hands on your thighs to support your weight. Bend your knees and lean a little forward with your upper body. Slowly roll up through the back, one vertebra at a time beginning with the lowest one and continuing up through your mid- and upper back. Your back should actually be curved like a shallow C. Your head should be aligned with your neck. Hold this stretch for a minute or two and then slowly roll back down to your semi-sitting position. Inhale when you curve up and exhale as you roll down.

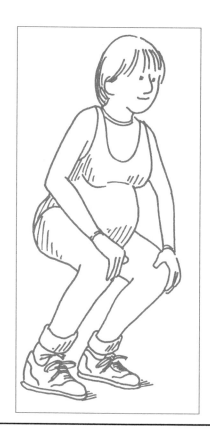

Squat

Squatting is a great exercise for preparing your perineum for delivery. Keep your back straight, open your legs, and move down. If you need a chair for support the first few times, grab the seat with both hands to steady yourself. Turn your feet out slightly and try to keep your heels flat on the floor. You may even want to roll up a towel or mat to put under your heels at first. You are stretching your inner thighs and you can increase the stretch by placing your elbows on top and pushing down very gently. Clasp your hands in front of you and try to hold this position for as long as you can.

Squatting loosens your pelvic joints while it strengthens your back and thigh muscles. A lot of squatting during the nine months leading up to delivery can actually protect your back and will ease back pain. As your baby grows bigger and bigger, just let your uterus rest right between your stretched-out thighs. Lengthen your back. Imagine a string pulling the very top of your head up to the ceiling.

Sit down on an exercise mat if you have one. Some moms find a carpeted floor just fine. Others want the cushion of a big, soft pillow or want to be up against a wall or something firm for back support.

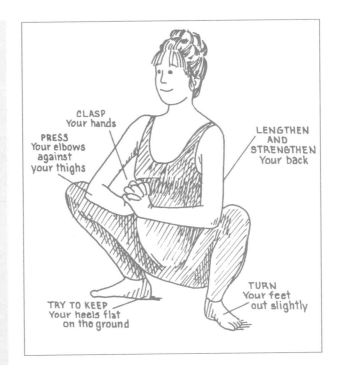

CLASP
Your hands

PRESS
Your elbows
against
your thighs

LENGTHEN
AND
STRENGTHEN
Your back

TRY TO KEEP
Your heels flat
on the ground

TURN
Your feet
out slightly

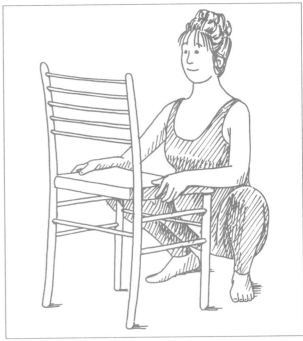

Sit to Stretch and Ease Strain

First, try sitting down on a mat or padded surface. With your legs in front of you, knees bent, and feet flat on the floor, clasp your hands in front of you. Keeping your arms straight, twist first to the left and then to the right of your bent knees. You'll be turning your shoulders to the right and then to the left and touching your clasped fingers to one side of your thighs and then to the other. An easy stretch, this movement actually strengthens the muscles of your back, hips, and abdomen, according to the American College of Obstetricians and Gynecologists (ACOG).

Cross Your Legs

Still seated, try crossing your legs in front of your body now in what is known as the semi-lotus position. Sit up as tall as you can. Put your hand under one backside cheek and lift it up and out. Then, reposition the other cheek as well so you are sitting squarely. Rest your hands on your knees easily. Relax. Breathe slowly in and out. Twist your body first to the right, allowing your left hand to grab your right knee as you move. Your right hand will move out to the right side and rest on the floor or mat to hold you steady during this trunk twist. Turn your head completely to the right and look around behind you. Change directions now.

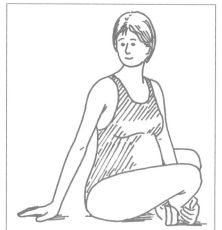
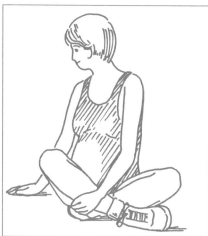
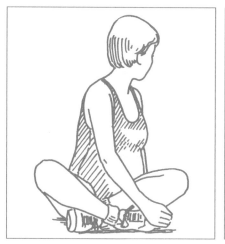
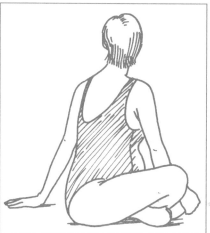

Ease Neck Strain

Stay seated and make sure your legs are comfortable. You don't want to cut off any circulation, so move a little if you feel your blood flow is being cut down even in the slightest. Let your knees flop outward and pull your legs in. Grab your ankles and put the soles of your feet together. Tilt your chin to your chest and clasp your hands at the back of your head with your elbows out. Press the back of your head toward your clasped hands.

Now, lift your chin so that your eyes are level and forward. Place your right hand on the top of your head and extend your left arm out to the side about eight to twelve inches from your body. Tilt your head toward the right. Your right ear is heading toward your right shoulder. Reach out with your left arm. Keep your eyes and your chin facing forward. Hold the position for up to ten seconds and breathe naturally. Repeat the movement on the other side.

Tailor Sit

Stay seated: with your back straight and your head held high, grab your ankles and bring the soles of your feet together directly in front of you. Pull your feet in as close to your body as you can. Your body is going to be more supple when you are pregnant because of the hormones circulating that are relaxing all your joints and ligaments, so this position may be easier than ever before in your life. Take hold of your ankles in this position and place your elbows and arms on your inner thighs. Press down slightly with your arms so that you push your thighs open wider.

Kneel Up and Stretch Out

Kneel up on your hands and knees. Make sure that your knees are about ten inches apart and your hands are just under your shoulders. You want to create the effect of a steady, sturdy table with your kneeling body and flat back. Keep your spine straight from head to tailbone as you begin. Now, curl your back up just as a cat might do when angry. Stretch way up and let your head drop between your shoulders. Now, let your spine slowly curl back down and lift your chin and head up in the opposite direction. In a rocking motion, repeat three or four times.

Twist Like a Cat

Stay in the kneeling position: try twisting from side to side, moving your head around to look at your heels, first to the left and then to the right. Exhale and turn back to the center. Inhale and twist in the opposite direction. Rest back and breathe deeply.

Reach Out

Still kneeling up on all fours, exhale and stretch your right hand forward while your left leg moves straight out in back. Feel them pull away from your body in either direction. You may lose your balance, so take this slowly. Push back with your heel flat while your toes remain pointed down. Stretch. Reach with your fingertips. Let your head hang loose. Bring hand and foot back in and relax. Do the other side, exhaling before each lift.

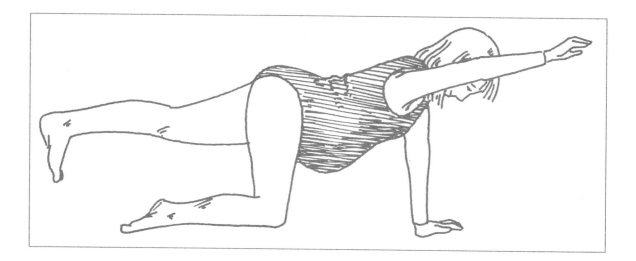

Sit Back on Your Heels and Reach Out . . . Relax

While you are still on the floor on all fours, slowly begin to sit back on your heels, curling your backside down until it is resting on the back of your calves. Tuck your head down and face into your bent knees while you stretch your arms out straight along the floor in front of you. Breathe in and out slowly. Reach out with your fingertips. Relax. Your belly should be resting easily between your thighs. Hold this stretched-out position for a few minutes before curling back up on all fours. Repeat three or four times.

Tone Your Pelvis

Kneel with your elbows on the floor, your chin resting on your hands, and your buttocks up in the air. This kind of knee-to-chest position allows your uterus to fall away from its pressing position on the pelvic floor. With your knees spread and your head still quietly resting on your crossed arms, tighten the muscles along your vagina and your rectum. Contract for a few seconds and then release. Repeat three to four times.

Put Your Back Against a Wall

Although it sounds easy, this exercise actually takes some stamina and will help strengthen your back, torso, and upper body. Stand with your upper back leaning against a smooth wall while your feet are firmly planted but about ten to twelve inches out. Lean the lower section of your spine into the wall. You'll feel the stress in your thighs. But do push back. Hold the position and count to ten. Rest. Repeat ten times.

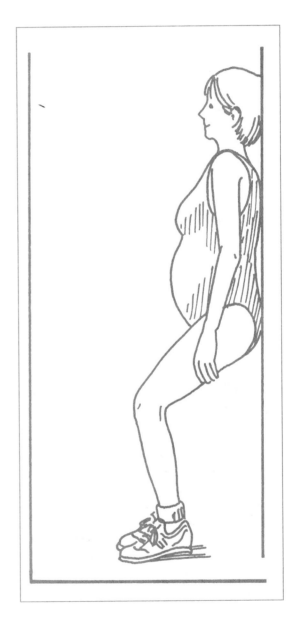

Lift Your Legs

Start out by kneeling on all fours once again. Your hands should be just beneath your shoulders for support. Knees are about ten inches apart. Keeping your hands flat and firmly planted on the floor or mat, lift your left knee and foot together in one motion out to the side of your body and then down again. You'll be trying to redistribute your weight so your arms remain steady and the right side of your body is still during these swings. Next, lift this bent left leg out to the back and drop it down to touch lightly on the mat. Use your hip to make this movement. Keep your spine steady. Lift to the side and back again. Repeat three to four times. Then, work your right leg in the same way.

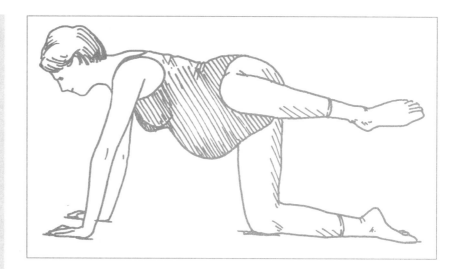

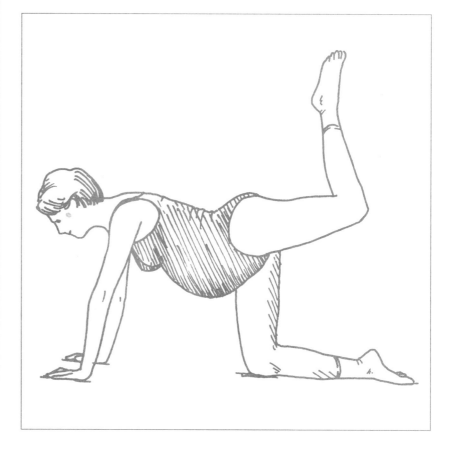

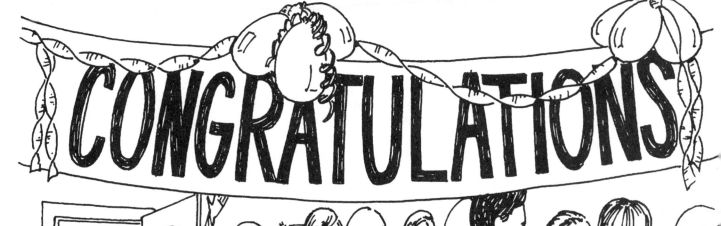

MONTH THREE

Pee-ing into little cups like a pro,
Getting weighed, measured, poked, prodded,
Telling others that, "Yes, it's true. . . ."
Some days, your smile says it all.

TO DO THIS MONTH

- ☐ *Tell people your good news.*
- ☐ *Steal time for yourself (even ten minutes a day!).*
- ☐ *Talk about tests with your doctor.*
- ☐ *Don't worry about your weight.*
- ☐ *Take a good look in your medicine cabinet.*
- ☐ *Go bra shopping.*

A tlanta pediatrician Sandy Matthews claims that women adapt to pregnancy in different ways. For more than thirty years, he's watched thousands of expectant moms in his busy practice and he likes to wax theoretically. "I like to think of living in a pregnant state in the same vein as learning to ride a bicycle," he insists. "When you first got up on that bicycle seat, you felt a little shaky. Maybe you fell off. But, you kept climbing back up to try it again because that new sensation was exhilaratingly different. Finally, then, you started speeding along. It was a unique talent or ability that you had all along."

What Are You Feeling Emotionally?

Bike riding on a bumpy, rut-filled road is no easy task. Neither is being pregnant. Be careful. Eat this. Don't drink that. Be aware of certain signs. How could you even consider doing that?!! By twelve weeks, you have reached a point still fraught with all those annoying first-trimester symptoms and concerns, but rest assured, there is an end in sight. You are up and riding. It's going to get smoother.

- Are you anxious to tell everyone that yes, you are pregnant?
- Aren't you amazed to think that right now, at this point in time, you are carrying an unborn baby that looks quite human? Although the head is still disproportionately large for the size of the two-inch body, imagine those little fingernails and toenails growing now.
- Is your mate's behavior annoying or worrisome? (Pssst . . . Turning yourself into a mother . . . even if this isn't your first child . . . is a monumental maturing process. During pregnancy, many couples complicate the transition to parenthood by worrying constantly and evaluating each other. Even during the happiest of pregnancies, fear of the unknown can dominate. You and your partner are bound to have mixed feelings. The elation about the news that you both may have experienced months ago could be clouded with concerns now. Talk about it. Don't fume in silence. Don't brood. Get out. Go on a date away from your home.

You both need a little romance even if your stomach is still lurching. The food will be less important than the honest conversation.

- Have you been preoccupied with strange, unexplainable side effects? Get the answers to all your questions. Don't ever fall for the line that you are reading or worrying too much for your own good. Those days of keeping patients in the dark are gone. Have you fantasized that your headaches point to nothing other than a brain tumor? Do you suspect that your baby has some dread genetic disease? Are you frightened that the testing your practitioner has scheduled for the coming weeks may cause a miscarriage? Speak up, and if you don't get the answer you need, consider switching to an expert who will be more forthcoming. Remember: you are not crazy. You are not paranoid. You are not anything but pregnant.

Oh Baby . . . Inside Secrets Now

- Your uterus is beginning to grow and stretch. There is plenty of room for the fetus to float in his or her warm, watery comfort zone while attached to the umbilical cord. Picture an astronaut, suggests well-known expert Virginia Apgar, M.D. "With his graceful, weightless movements, his life-support system and the perils of his existence, one scientist nicknamed him an 'intronaut.'"

- Because fetal muscles and nerves are working together, your baby starts moving at first tentatively, then more seriously, deliberately, and vigorously by month's end. Dr. Apgar says that the fetus kicks, swims, twists, turns around, pivots, and even somersaults. "He can move his thumb in opposition to his fingers. He can open his mouth, swallow, inhale and exhale, curl his toes, bend his wrist and his waist and make a fist. In fact," she states, "an unborn baby can perform many maneuvers in his watery environment five months before his birth that he will not be able to duplicate again until several months after his birth."

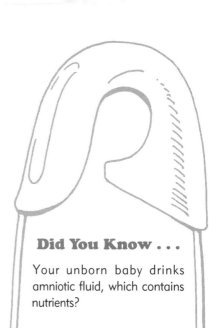

Did You Know . . .

Your unborn baby drinks amniotic fluid, which contains nutrients?

The top of your womb should be stretching up above your pubic bone this month?

You have more blood in your body now?

- You can't feel all this movement in your unborn baby yet. Just wait until next month.
- Facial features are becoming more pronounced, more human, more attractive. He or she looks like someone in your own family now. Eyes are closer together. Eyelids have grown long enough to shut now and they will stay shut until the last trimester.
- Vocal cords are in place but making sounds isn't possible.
- Sucking is now possible. Taste buds and saliva glands develop. Soon, when swallowing is developed, the baby will drink amniotic fluid into a newly formed stomach. The amniotic fluid contains nutrients that help the fetus grow. In fact, drinking helps those tiny kidneys to begin processing and later, the fetus will urinate. Don't worry. Fetal urine is quite sterile and goes directly back into the amniotic fluid.
- A fetus may inhale some of the amniotic fluid, but there is no danger of drowning. Your unborn baby isn't breathing— that won't happen until he sees the light of day, even though breathing motions can be detected. All of the oxygen is being supplied by you via the umbilical cord.
- Sex organs are evident, but even the most skillful ultrasound operator can't always be certain to catch the fetal pose you need to see for yourself.
- Skin is so thin that it is transparent. You can see the blood vessel network clearly.
- Your baby looks hairy because of a covering of soft down called *lanugo*.
- The heart is beating twice as fast as yours and you may be able to hear it now. A Doppler device, which is a combination of ultrasound and amplifier, can sometimes pick up this wonderful sound as early as 10 or 12 weeks but by the 18th week, you are more certain of catching this music to your ears.
- Your unborn baby has earlobes.
- Weight is approximately $5/8$ of an ounce, or 18 grams. Length is about 9 centimeters at the end of month three.

Let's Get Physical

Take It Easy Now . . . Take Care of Yourself

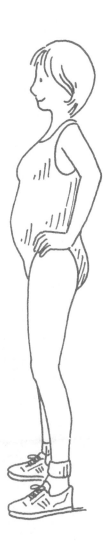

- Put your finger just above your pubic bone. That's where the top of your womb is already. Isn't it amazing how this little being you have yet to meet could be changing your very shape?
- Weight gain varies tremendously, especially during this first trimester. If you haven't had morning sickness, making it hard to eat, $2^{1}/_{2}$ pounds growth puts you on target. Many women put on much more than this meager beginning, however, and these pounds are quite legitimate. After all, you are growing a new life. The waistband on your slacks, jeans, and skirts may feel snug. Take time to treat yourself to something new to wear that won't tug or make you feel as if you have eaten too much.
- Investigate prenatal exercise classes in your area. If you are uncertain where to begin, ask the experts in your doctor or midwife's office. Pick up flyers, booklets, or handouts about local classes being held in hospitals, private studios, or sports clubs. Not only will you be taking good care of your body, but also you may be able to network and commiserate with other pregnant women.
- Take stock of your daily diet. Are you eating five servings of fruits and vegetables every day? Are you taking your vitamins? Folic acid is absolutely essential to the health of your unborn baby. If you are constipated, drink more water. If you are still suffering from morning sickness, take heart. Most women's stomachs settle down in the second trimester. You are almost there.
- Be kind to yourself. Stop racing and expecting a completed to-do list at the end of your day. Schedule time for naps. Your lungs, kidneys, and heart are all working harder than ever because of the increased volume of blood circulating in your body.

Get the Most Out of Monthly Check-Ups

You've probably been to visit your doctor or midwife's office at least twice by now. Perhaps you've settled into a happy routine and look forward to these updates. However,

- Are you comfortable?
- Are you getting all your questions answered?
- Have you settled any concerns about insurance, payments, managed care plans, and other frustrating paperwork problems?

You may have special concerns and requests. For instance, what is this doctor's cesarean rate? What is her approach to pain medication during labor and delivery? Write down your questions beforehand. Do your homework. Ask other mothers, friends, and relatives for inside tips on making your pregnancy go as smoothly as possible. And, remember, your doctor or midwife is a professional who is working for you. You have hired this individual and you should never feel belittled or feel childish in his or her presence. You have more power than you think.

Don't Forget to Ask

- At which hospital or birthing center will you give birth? Don't assume you know. Find out and schedule a visit so you can look around and ask questions. Most hospitals offer tours of the nursery, labor and delivery rooms, as well as where you'll be after the baby is born.
- What kind of special services or privileges exist for childbirth? Many hospitals are actually courting obstetrical and maternity business and offer private suites, champagne dinners, and various birthing options to make your stay both comfortable and safe.
- What kind of emergency or special neonatal departments does the hospital have? Not every medical facility offers

neonatal intensive care for babies born prematurely or with grave problems. Find out what your doctor plans to do if any of your worst nightmares should come true. For more information about special neonatal options, see Month Seven.

- How does your doctor feel about weight gain? A strict approach might make you feel guilty, inadequate, or downright fat later. You want to stay healthy, regain your shape soon after birth, and gain exactly what you need to nourish a healthy baby, but you also want to maintain a strong self-image.

- If your doctor is in a group practice, will you be able to meet and visit with every other member? You don't want to meet a stranger when you are in labor.

Make a Personal Impression

Think about the nurses and administrative staff in the doctor's office you have met by now. Which ones are your favorites? Do you know their names? Introduce yourself next time and take a minute to jot down the name so you can have it for the next visit or the next time you call and end up speaking with someone on the phone besides your doctor. Make these relationships personal and you will gain more from the encounters. In fact, the doctor's secretary or office manager may be key to helping you through a myriad of obstacles.

In Your Doctor's Bag of Tools and Tests

Testing seems to be the name of the game in modern pregnancies. Not only is your doctor making sure that the unborn baby is growing normally, but also a variety of other concerns are explored. No test is foolproof, of course, but early warnings of trouble are well worth your discomfort or anxiety. Some tests, such as amniocentesis and the alpha-fetoprotein (AFP), may be scheduled early in your second trimester.

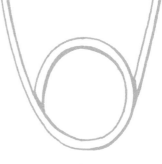

Soooo . . . Other Pregnant Women Have These Symptoms, Too:

- Tender breasts
- Fatigue
- Occasional dizziness
- Frequent urination
- Nausea
- Insomnia
- Constipation
- Indigestion
- Stomach as well as intestinal gas
- Runny nose
- Headaches
- Vaginal discharge
- Signs of varicose veins
- Cravings for strange foods; aversions to old favorites
- Weird changes in skin and hair

You Are Going to Urinate into Little Cups All the Time!

Regular samples of urine taken during office visits will show not only that you are pregnant but also the levels of sugar, protein, and other substances in your body. Signs of urinary infection can also be detected. Traces of sugar can be a sign of diabetes and too much protein could mean that your kidneys aren't working properly. Later, protein in your urine is a warning of a rare, but serious complication, called *preeclampsia* or pregnancy-induced high blood pressure. The most important substance in your urine right now is human chorionic gonadtropin, or HCG, which is produced by the embryo as it becomes attached to your uterus. A hormone, HCG streams into your circulation, moves through your kidneys, and is later excreted through your kidneys. In your third trimester, HCG levels dissipate.

A Pap Smear Will Rule Out Cancer

If you've been having regular gynecological check-ups, you probably already know that your doctor will scrape your cervix during an internal examination to test cells for signs of cancer. When you are pregnant, pap smear results can be confusing because of the biochemical changes in your body. If the test turns up positive the first time, a second pap smear may be required for another opinion. Relax. Mention your concerns to your doctor. The American College of Obstetricians and Gynecologists now requires all women to have a pap test within three months of pregnancy.

You'll Be Giving Blood Once, Twice, and Perhaps Even More Often

The amount of blood in your body actually increases when you are pregnant. In fact, the fluid portion goes up by approximately 40 percent. Meanwhile, your red blood cell count may rise by about 20 percent. This disparity—the increase in plasma but not quite as much in red blood cells—can cause anemia. Blood testing will check for anemia, or lack of iron, as well as sexually transmitted diseases. Blood tests also determine whether or not you are immune to German measles or rubella. Even if you can't remember if you had it

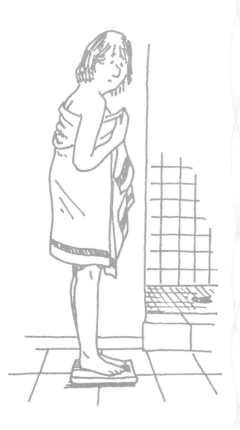

A Doctor's Note:
Weigh Yourself Only on Fridays!

Pregnancy is really a high cholesterol state brought on by your hormones. Some doctors feel that an excess weight gain during these nine months can be the start of arterio sclerotic problems. That's why you really need to define what you mean by excess weight. Four to five pounds a month is not an excessive amount to gain, but twelve pounds can be. If you were left alone without any advice and you ate a well-balanced, constant diet, you would gain one-half of your weight in the first six months and the second half in the last three months. So when I see a pregnant patient with excess weight gain in the first and second trimester, I suspect they will double their weight in the last trimester. Someone who has gained ten pounds a month may begin to gain twenty pounds a month. All pregnant women say they are going to lose weight in the postpartum period, but it is the most difficult thing to do right after birth. What most women should aim for is a gain of twenty to twenty-five pounds, an amount that can be lost at delivery. You really don't have to sacrifice your vanity to have a baby. This is what I do with my patients. When they tell me they haven't eaten anything in spite of a ten-pound gain, I ask them to write down their diets for one week. They all lose weight when they return to my office.

Even if you aren't pregnant, here's a tip: Weigh yourself only on Friday. Most of us binge on Saturday or Sunday. Then you can watch your eating habits the rest of the week to see what happens.

—Howard Berk, M.D.

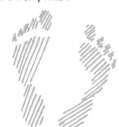

or not, your blood will tell the truth. German measles or rubella can cause birth defects, especially if you contract the infection during the first trimester. Babies whose mothers contracted rubella early in pregnancy can end up with cataracts (eye problems), heart defects, and deafness. A majority of women have been exposed to the rubella virus or have been vaccinated against it before becoming pregnant, however. Immunity lasts a lifetime. By the end of the first trimester, the risk to your unborn baby is smaller.

Testing also tells the doctor your blood type as well as your rhesus, or Rh, factor. Your blood belongs to one of four major groups: A, B, AB, or O. Your blood is also rhesus (Rh) positive or rhesus (Rh) negative. The word *rhesus* comes from the rhesus monkeys that were used in the first laboratory experiments with red blood cells. If you are Rh negative and your unborn baby is positive, you could have complications. Only women who are negative need to be concerned, in fact. If an Rh-negative mom's blood somehow combines with the baby's Rh-positive blood, her immune system may try to fight off the baby as an intruder, causing prenatal death or brain damage in the baby. In essence, mother and baby are incompatible. You'll be screened for signs of these antibodies and given an injection of an anti-Rh immunoglobuin (Rhogam) when you reach the twenty-eighth week of pregnancy. The injections stop your immune system from creating antibodies that could hurt your baby.

Blood tests can also indicate inherited anemia. For example, the sickle cell trait can be determined for African or Indian couples who must be particularly sensitive to this situation. Thalassemia can be a problem for families of Mediterranean, Middle East, or Far East origins.

Your Blood Pressure Is Going to Be Checked Regularly

The doctor, midwife, or nurse assistant will be measuring your blood pressure at each visit. To take your blood pressure your practitioner will use a stethoscope and a device, called a *sphygmomanometer*, that has an inflatable cuff that wraps around your arm and a pressure gauge. The reading obtained will consist of two numbers separated by a slash mark. You may hear it referred to as 120 over 70, normal, or 140 over 90, which is high and a reason to worry. The first number, known as *systolic pressure*, is the pressure of your arteries as your heart contracts. The second number, *diastolic pressure*, is being measured when your heart is relaxed in between contractions.

Because you are pregnant, your blood pressure may be a little lower than normal. Meanwhile, a rise in blood pressure can alert the doctor to several problems, including preeclampsia. A slight rise in blood pressure doesn't mean you have developed hypertension or a chronic condition. Just sitting there waiting in the doctor's office, anticipating the fact that you will be weighed, measured, poked, and prodded can make your blood pressure rise. If you are anxious about test results, your concern can also cause a temporary rise. So can exercise, stress, or even normal activity. Make sure you are told what your blood pressure is. It's always on your chart, so if you have forgotten to ask, take a look.

You'll Be Hopping on the Scale at Each Visit

Getting weighed is routine fare for these regular pregnancy check-ups. Be prepared to see the numbers go up consistently. Don't make yourself depressed or crazy about your gain, however. Keep your focus on a healthy baby and a healthy pregnancy, not on some preconceived chart of perfect pounds gained and lost.

Ultrasound Waves Can Create a Picture of Your Unborn Baby

Your practitioner may choose to order ultrasound to get a closer look at the progress inside your uterus. The picture, or *sonogram*, is obtained when high-frequency sound waves, which you can't hear, are passed over your growing uterus with a little hand-held machine called a *transducer*. These waves penetrate your body, send back a living, moving image of the tiny being inside, and transmit the picture to a computer or television screen. You can "see" the baby weeks before the heartbeat can even be heard or detected. Ultrasounds do not rely on radiation and absolutely no side effects have ever been found. Both kids and moms are safe. Don't forget to ask for a copy of the picture. This marvelous piece of technology is now available in hospitals, clinics, testing centers, as well as doctor's offices.

The ultrasound is also used for diagnostic tests that can be performed as early as five weeks and will allow you to rest assured about a variety of factors: Is your baby growing steadily? Is he breathing? Is she moving? In fact, are you carrying a boy, a girl, or twins? How is your placenta positioned? What's the heart rate? Is there enough amniotic fluid? Certain birth defects can also be determined early in pregnancy. Placental abnormalities, an ectopic pregnancy, or other abnormalities of pregnancy can show up on an ultrasound. If you are experiencing any kind of unusual bleeding, an ultrasound is the best tool for aiding the doctor in a diagnosis.

Ultrasound Insight: *What Exactly Happens*

If you are scheduled for an ultrasound early in pregnancy before week 20, for instance, the doctor may ask you to drink plenty of water before you arrive. Sound waves or beams actually need fluid for better conduction. That can translate into three or four glasses up to an hour before appointment time without freedom to go to the bathroom. (Your bladder control will get a workout on ultrasound days!) A full bladder helps the technician create the perfect picture of your uterus. The pelvic organs are easier to see, too, because the bladder actually pushes your bowel up and out of the way. Later in pregnancy, drinking up to the breaking point may not be necessary before an ultrasound because the enlarged uterus sits right on top of your pubic bone and amniotic fluid helps the process go smoother.

Be forewarned that there are two types of ultrasound scans: the transabdominal, or across the abdomen, and the transvaginal, or directly into your vagina. In very early pregnancy, the technician may opt for the vaginal approach, which means that the transducer will be inserted into your vagina. Be sure to ask which one you will be having so you aren't surprised. Abdominal ultrasounds are the most common.

You will climb up on the table and be asked to pull up your shirt or hospital gown to expose the lower part of your abdomen, from the bottom of your rib cage to your pelvis. Then, a thin application of paste, jelly, or oil will be spread over the skin on your abdomen to improve the contact between the transducer and the machine recording the sound waves. The technician will pass the transducer back and forth across your abdomen, sending and receiving the waves that help create the image you'll see on the screen. Don't let your husband miss this appointment. The chance to see your developing baby moving, sucking a thumb, kicking, turning, twisting inside your womb can be a life-changing experience.

After twenty years of use, ultrasounds are still not always considered routine in the United States even though they have become absolutely everyday adventures in pregnancy. Outside U.S. borders, doctors often schedule pregnant women for a minimum of two ultrasounds. Your doctor may need some kind of indication or reason to order an ultrasound and the desire to know if you are carrying a boy or a girl is not a good enough one. The test costs anywhere from $200 to $500, but it's not possible to schedule one on your own. If you think you would be more comfortable knowing everything is safe and your baby is behaving normally on an ultrasound, even though your doctor has not ordered one, simply explain your anxiety. Perhaps your fears could be reason enough to order the test.

Can Ultrasounds Ever Give Misleading Information?

Occasionally, parents wonder about the accuracy of the information obtained from an ultrasound. "Is the baby really a boy?" If the sonogram indicates a due date that seems wrong, you might question, "Could I possibly have dated the start of my pregnancy incorrectly?" Experts say that if the ultrasound is done at sixteen weeks and beyond, results are pretty accurate, although the equipment and the skill of the technician are factors to be considered. When an ultrasound is scheduled during the first trimester (in the first twelve weeks of your pregnancy), the accuracy drops a bit. A very clear image must be obtained for the ultrasound to determine whether you are expecting a boy or a girl, for instance. This may be more difficult to see in the early stages. Don't worry, most technicians won't say for certain unless they are absolutely certain. When dating the length of a pregnancy, the ultrasound technician can be accurate within a few days. Ultrasounds also date your pregnancy from the point of conception, which is a few days different from the point of your last period.

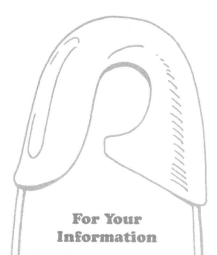

For Your Information

According to a study conducted by psychologist Erling Anderson of the University of Iowa, heart surgery patients who have prepared for surgery by becoming more knowledgeable about the procedure report less fear and have an easier recovery period. Pregnancy and childbirth are no different. "Information per se is not inherently reassuring," Dr. Anderson once stated. "But it is necessary because people can use it to plan ways to deal with what's happening."

You May Be Confronted with a CVS Test

CVS stands for *chorionic villus sampling*. This is a test that can be done during the first trimester if your doctor is worried about chromosome or biochemical abnormalities in the unborn baby. An ultrasound will be used to guide a soft tube to the tiny chorionic villi, which surround the embryo. Then, a sample, or biopsy, of the chorion is obtained and the cells are tested. CVS can be performed several weeks before amniocentesis, a test that is not considered accurate until you are nearly into your second trimester. Amniocentesis testing results can take up to ten days to obtain while CVS conclusions are drawn quicker. The CVS cytologist, or cell specialist, does not need to prepare a culture but can examine the fresh cells right away. Some answers can be obtained within forty-eight hours after a CVS. An early diagnosis of Down's syndrome, for instance, may be important for some couples to know. If there is a history of genetic defects in your family, this may also be a very good reason to go for the CVS.

If you are being offered the option of a CVS, there are several issues of safety and procedure you should be sure to bring up with your doctor. The chance of miscarriage from CVS is up to 30 percent, according to some experts. If your pregnancy is a hard-won state of being and you spent months or even years reaching this point in your first trimester, you may not want to risk losing your baby now. Speak up and have your doctor research the very latest statistics as well as methods. Keep in mind these factors, too:

- CVS is not always accurate. The exact spot where the technician removes the cell sampling from the chorion can be critical. In some cases, cells have been inaccurately taken from the mother's own tissue, which would offer no indication of the health of the unborn baby. Also, some abnormalities in chorionic tissues do not always show up in the fetus. Ask for clarification or a second opinion of any negative CVS report before you decide on any course of action in your pregnancy.
- Find out which CVS method will be used on you. CVS relies on an ultrasound machine to guide the tube inside you, but the catheter can be inserted either through your vagina or

Certificate of Birth

Ask Good Questions

This is an art you are going to master . . . now and throughout your mothering adventure. Don't be shy. The better you get at asking questions, the easier it will be to obtain the information you need.

- Use open-ended questions. Begin with who, what, when, where, and how. If you use why as an opener, you may put your doctor on the defensive.

- Tone of voice is critical. If you are preoccupied, hungry, furious, frustrated, or too tired to think straight, you are not going to be able to ask good questions or hear answers clearly.

- Face the person to whom you are speaking. If you are asking questions when you are up on the examining table and your doctor's head is not even in your line of vision, you are not going to be able to have a proper discussion.

- Get clarification for anything you don't understand.

- Be specific. What exactly does your doctor mean? Are you being bombarded by medical terms you don't understand? Don't worry about appearing stupid. Take it slow. If a word is unclear, politely ask for an explanation. If the issue of a particular test comes up, ask exactly what he intends to find out from the results of the procedure. Reserve the right to ask additional questions later, too.

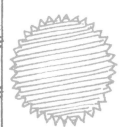

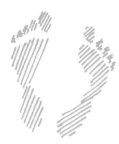

directly down through your abdomen in a method called *transabdominal.* If your doctor has not discussed the difference between the two, don't schedule the test until you get a full report. Published research doesn't show any real differences between the two, so pick your physician's brain about his preferences.

Your Legs, Ankles, and Hands Will Be Checked for Swelling

When you are up on the examining table during a regular prenatal check-up, you should not be surprised to see the doctor or midwife gently poke the skin on your lower legs, your ankles, and your hands. In pregnancy lots of women develop fluid buildup, but excessive swelling could mean the development of high blood pressure or preeclampsia.

Your Abdomen Will Be Gently Pushed, Probed, and Measured

An old-fashioned, but remarkably accurate, clue to how your pregnancy is progressing is to have your doctor or nurse-midwife gently feel for the top of your womb. A tape measure is also an option because your uterus grows at a steady rate, or three centimeters per month, until it pushes up above your belly button (at twenty weeks) and reaches just below your rib cage.

Obstetrician Howard Shapiro says that you can check this growth on your own starting at the end of the first trimester. Go to the bathroom and empty your bladder completely. Then lie down on a hard, flat surface and put your hand just above your pubic bone. If you think you are at least twelve weeks pregnant, then you should be able to feel the uterus. If you sense that your uterus is growing much faster than is considered normal, your hunch could indicate that you are carrying twins or at least a very large baby. In the last trimester, your tape measure should stretch out to nearly thirty-six centimeters of growth. However, this height may suddenly drop in the last few weeks as your baby begins his escape down and out into the real world through your pelvis.

Inside Your Medicine Chest

Your first and last trimesters are the most critical periods of development for your baby. Yet, making expectant mothers anxious about medication has only recently been considered appropriate. According to Dr. Howard Berk, new scientific evidence supports his belief that, "Anything you can buy over the counter, you can take when you are pregnant." If there is a question, consult with your practitioner. In the meantime, don't worry, says Berk. You don't need to live in fear of every move you make or every burp you take.

The Food and Drug Administration (FDA) continues to study the issue of medications during pregnancy. If you are interested in doing your own research about drugs during pregnancy and have access to the Internet, you might want to visit the Web site called MedicineNet, State of the Art Medical Information (http://medicinenet.com).

Good Advice from the FDA

All over-the-counter drugs are required to carry the warning label: "As with any drug, if you are pregnant or nursing, seek the advice of a health professional before using this product." There are five FDA categories of safety, from A (safest) to X (not a good idea at all). Whether you need to take a regular antibiotic, an anti-epileptic drug for seizures, or use an asthma inhaler for hay fever season, you should be able to understand the degree of safety. Not all drugs have been assigned one of these lettered categories and drug manufacturers are not legally bound to publicize FDA pronouncements about a particular medicine. However, these definitions are important to know:

- **A** Controlled studies in women fail to demonstrate a risk to the fetus in the first trimester; there is no evidence of risk in later trimesters; and the possibility of fetal harm appears remote.

- **B** Either animal reproduction studies have not demonstrated a fetal risk, but there are no controlled studies in pregnant

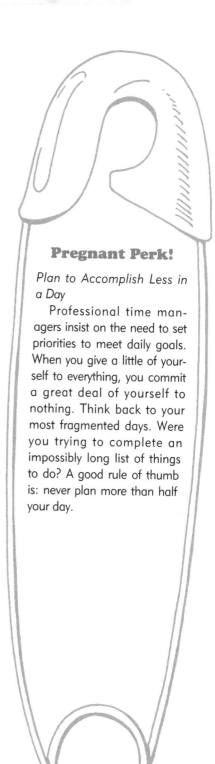

Pregnant Perk!

Plan to Accomplish Less in a Day

Professional time managers insist on the need to set priorities to meet daily goals. When you give a little of yourself to everything, you commit a great deal of yourself to nothing. Think back to your most fragmented days. Were you trying to complete an impossibly long list of things to do? A good rule of thumb is: never plan more than half your day.

women in the first trimester and there is no evidence of a risk in later trimesters.

- **C** Either studies in animals have revealed adverse effects on the fetus (teratogenic, embryocidal, or other) and there are no controlled studies in women, or studies in women and animals are not available. The drug should be given only if the potential benefit justifies the potential risk to the fetus.

- **D** There is positive evidence of human fetal risk, but the benefits from use in pregnant women may be acceptable despite the risk—for example, if the drug is needed for a life-threatening situation or for a serious disease for which safer drugs cannot be used or are ineffective.

- **X** Studies in animals or human beings have demonstrated fetal abnormalities, or there is evidence of fetal risk based on human experience or both, and the risk of the use of the drug in pregnant women clearly outweighs any of the benefits. The drug is contraindicated in women who are or may become pregnant.

RX: Take This Harmful Hit List Seriously

The American Academy of Obstetricians and Gynecologists (ACOG) suggests that these categories of substances, or teratogens, should be red flags in your pregnant life. Be sure to speak with your practitioner about:

- Alcohol
- Androgens (used to treat endometriosis)
- Anticoagulants (to prevent blood clotting)
- Antithyroids (for people with overactive thyroids)
- Anticonvulsants (for seizure disorders or irregular heartbeats)

- Aspirin or any tablet containing salicylate (for pain relief) during the last three weeks because of bleeding complications not because it will cause any congenital malformations.
- Chemotherapeutic drugs (used to treat cancer and skin diseases)
- Diethylstilbestrol (once used to treat premature labor and miscarriage; still prescribed for menstrual problems, symptoms of menopause, and breast cancer)
- Isotreinoin (also known as Accutane, prescribed for cystic acne)
- Lead (found in industrial situations and in paints)
- Lithium (used for treatment of depression)
- Organic mercury (can be exposed to it via contaminated foods)
- Streptomycin (antibiotic used for tuberculosis)
- Tetracycline (antibiotic used for a wide variety of infections)
- Thalidomide (once prescribed as a sleep aid and sedative)
- X-ray (used to treat cancer in radiation treatments)

Just an Aspirin?

Sure. Aspirin was once considered a problem, but unless you are in your last three weeks, it's no longer considered dangerous. Connecticut obstetrician-gynecologist and author Howard Shapiro states, "Almost all chemical substances can cross the placenta and become concentrated in the fetus. Whether or not a drug causes harm depends on many factors, including the genetic makeup of the mother and fetus, the specific chemical structure of the drug, the month of pregnancy in which the drug is used, and the total dose." Actually the placenta is a filter that has the ability to screen out substances above a certain size. Small molecules get through and others don't. That's why if you have the flu, the flu won't affect the baby. Yet, small viruses like herpes and chicken pox can get through. This filtering process protects your baby.

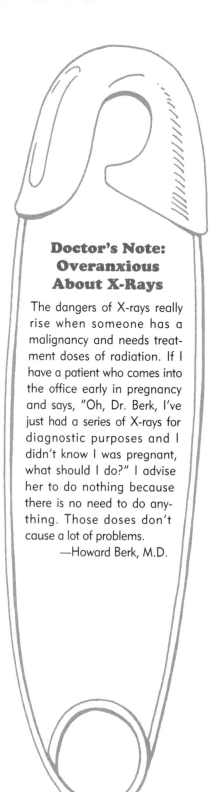

Doctor's Note: Overanxious About X-Rays

The dangers of X-rays really rise when someone has a malignancy and needs treatment doses of radiation. If I have a patient who comes into the office early in pregnancy and says, "Oh, Dr. Berk, I've just had a series of X-rays for diagnostic purposes and I didn't know I was pregnant, what should I do?" I advise her to do nothing because there is no need to do anything. Those doses don't cause a lot of problems.

—Howard Berk, M.D.

Common Medication Questions

What should you take for a headache?

Aspirin is fine for most of your pregnancy. Avoid it in the last month. Tylenol or an analgesic based on acetaminophen are also recommended for headaches.

I have terrible allergies and can hardly breathe during the spring. Is there anything at all my doctor is going to be able to recommend?

Sometimes nasal stuffiness and symptoms that mimic allergies are actually side effects of early pregnancy. Research has been conducted on allergy medications and their safe use during pregnancy, but Dr. Berk insists that over-the-counter drugs will do no harm in pregnancy. If you are worried about antihistamines, which were once thought to be harmful in pregnancy, check with your practitioner.

If I develop an infection, are there any antibiotics safe for expectant moms?

Yes, pharmaceutical companies are coming up with new antibiotics all the time and a number of them are safe for pregnancy. According to Dr. Lauerson, "Natural and synthetic penicillins are the safest antibiotics to take during pregnancy," so if you are not allergic to these oldest weapons against infection, you are definitely in luck. If you do get sick, make sure that your obstetrician is aware of anything your family doctor or another specialist may be prescribing. Doctors need to work together as a team to treat you during this very special time of your life.

I have epilepsy and have been seizure free for several years thanks to my medication. Can I still take my antiepileptic drugs and deliver a healthy baby?

Many obstetricians and pharmacologists get very worried when you mention the words pregnancy and epilepsy in the same context. However, when you speak to an epileptologist (a doctor specializing in seizure treatment), the news is not all doom and gloom. Andrew Wilner, M.D., of The Neurology Foundation, Providence, RI, and author of *Epilepsy, 199 Answers*, explains, "Although medications can cause birth defects, they usually do not. The risk of birth defects in children to women with epilepsy is about 6 percent. That means there is a 94 percent chance there will be no birth defects." Dr. Wilner suggests that you sit down with your specialist and plan your pregnancy very carefully, making certain not to begin or stop taking any medications without serious consideration. "The risk of harm to you and your baby is probably greater if you have a convulsion than the risk to your baby from medication." He also explains that pregnancy is a good time to reevaluate the drugs you may be taking. Your body will be undergoing profound biochemical changes and you may even want to have the drug levels in your blood checked much more frequently than in your recent past. You really want to take "the least number of drugs at the lowest dosages to control your seizures."

The Stress Factor

Should You Be Worried About Being Worried?

While it's only natural to feel a certain amount of anxiety about all the unknowns of pregnancy, perhaps you sense that your level of unhealthy stress seems to be escalating week by week. Can this be affecting your unborn baby? Lauerson's advice should make you feel better already. A clinical professor of Obstetrics and Gynecology at New York Medical College, he explains, "Researchers have never uncovered any evidence that emotional ups

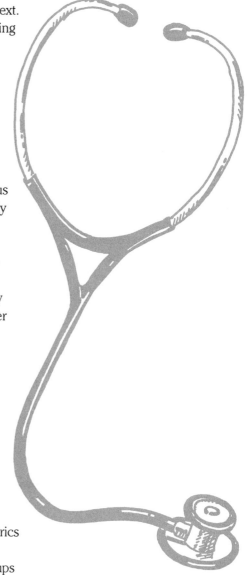

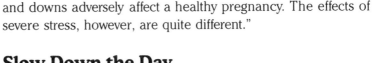

and downs adversely affect a healthy pregnancy. The effects of severe stress, however, are quite different."

Slow Down the Day

Give Your Body a Boost

Sometimes a speeded-up sense of inner timing can make you feel like racing through the day. Here are tips to put back some measure of control of your biology and your growing baby:

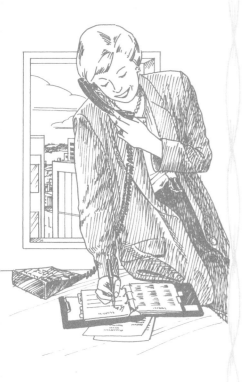

- Chronic stress is "like having one foot on the accelerator of a car with the other foot on the brake, we wind up stripping our gears," reports Reed Moskowitz, M.D., of New York University's Stress Disorders Services. Simply recognizing this connection between stress and your health is a step in the right direction.
- Researchers at Penn State found that women who pushed themselves to the limits, working till the end of their pregnancies in what they called "stand up" jobs were more likely to have placental problems, including areas of dead tissue in the placenta caused by impaired blood flow. Although babies did not show long-term mental or physical impairment, slowing down to a more leisurely pace turned out to be as important mentally as it was physically.

Good Idea: When Life Is Making You Feel Crazy . . .

Emotional Stress

If you are working or living under chronically stressful conditions, give yourself permission to seek support, advice, and professional counsel from your obstetrician. You're not being a wimp at all. You are actually protecting the life of your unborn baby. In 1990, a University of North Carolina study found that high levels of stress led to low-birth-weight babies and complications during pregnancy, such as hypertension, preeclampsia, and premature birth.

How can you define high stress? You are the best person to determine what sends you off the top of the stress scale and into unhealthy territory. If you are working outside your home in an environment that offers you little control but features high levels of emotional stress, then you probably know who you are. Look for ways to eliminate anxiety and you may even lessen your need for pain medication during labor and birth. Yale University experts discovered that if you exhibit high anxiety during pregnancy, you fall into the category of women who need the most medication.

Even if you can't come up with concrete ways to escape your stressful situation, experts like Dr. Moskowitz believe that your coping style can make a world of difference. Take a long look at your approach to this pregnancy. Which one of these personality types fits you best?

- *You create loving bonds*. You have a sense of humor. You anticipate conflicts and how they will make you feel. You consciously put off stresses you know you aren't ready to handle. You know how to turn your own socially unacceptable behavior into something useful. For example, an overeater might "harness her basic eating drive into a career as a gourmet chef." Turn anxiety and curiosity about the entire pregnancy process into a very personal research project.
- *You alienate people*. You deny needing help and don't take responsibility for your actions. You tend to block out your emotions, often unconsciously. You are impulsive in destructive ways. Self-righteous, you project feelings onto others that aren't there. Perhaps you are accusing your husband of not caring enough about the pregnancy or not planning far enough ahead for the birth. You turn minor aches into major diseases or baby disasters.

"The differences between these two coping styles is astounding," according to Dr. Moskowitz. See where you fit in and work to change the way you handle stress.

Emergency Business

Most pregnancies have happy endings. Yet, you might feel that everything about your pregnancy can be a cause for worry on occasion. Your body may not feel familiar, so why shouldn't creepy symptoms keep you up at night? If you've been placed into a high-risk category because of a combination of factors, then even the simplest, yet unusual, symptoms can be frightening. Never hesitate to call your doctor or midwife about anything. No question is too silly to ask. No sensation is too mild to mention. Here are just some of the factors that may have placed you into a high-risk situation and will make your case even more important for your practitioner to watch closely.

Emergencies can happen any time during a pregnancy, but knowing that you are in a high-risk situation is important for both you and your physician to take into consideration. Go over this list of potential reasons for considering your pregnancy high risk. These are certainly issues you have already discussed with your medical team, but just in case, make a note of any that fit your situation.

- Is there a history of diabetes in your family? In fact, do you have diabetes?
- High blood pressure?
- Heart problems?
- Tuberculosis?
- Asthma and/or allergies?
- Thyroid disorder?
- Any uterine or pelvic abnormalities? Fibroid tumors? Ovarian cysts?
- Have you been diagnosed with a sexually transmitted disease?
- Does your family's genetic history place you in a high-risk category, too?
- Your age is a factor and you are considered high risk. Are you a teenager or over thirty-five?
- Did you experience a problem giving birth or during a previous pregnancy? A miscarriage? Stillbirth? Premature birth? Cesarean section?

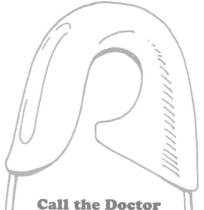

I Was Wondering . . .

Does bleeding in the first trimester always mean that a miscarriage is imminent?

Not always. However, vaginal bleeding is often the first sign of an impending miscarriage, so you have every reason to worry if you notice spots of blood on your underpants. Yes, of course, those stains can be enough to make your heart drop straight through the floor. Yet, staining does not always indicate the beginning of the end of your pregnancy and more than 20 percent of women who bleed early in pregnancy go on to deliver healthy babies. Sometimes, if the spotting occurs very early in those first days of pregnancy, the blood is just a sign of implantation indicating that the fertilized egg is attaching itself to the lining of your uterus. If you have had sex with your mate, a bit of blood can be caused by the contact during intercourse.

Bleeding, in fact, is not dangerous when it comes from your cervix. If the bleeding is from your uterus, it is more serious. Your doctor may even ask if it is bright red blood or darker in color. A dark blood stain is a sign of bleeding that occurred several days before. If your bleeding is bright red and you also have low back pain and abdominal cramping, call your doctor immediately.

If you have children already, you are more likely to experience some bleeding. However, bleeding a bit during the same time of the month that you would have expected to be getting your period is not normal during pregnancy. If you notice blood, call your doctor, lie down (preferably on your left side), and try not to panic. Bleeding can start and stop on its own. If the bleeding is slight and stops on its own, your chances of delivering a healthy baby are fine. More than one instance of bleeding or prolonged bleeding during the first trimester should put you and your doctor on edge, however. Statistics on miscarriage differ, but the American College of Obstetricians and Gynecologists (ACOG) reports that 15 to 20 percent of all pregnancies end in miscarriage in the first thirteen weeks. Your risk of miscarriage decreases dramatically after the first trimester, and after hearing your baby's heartbeat, that risk drops even further to about 3 percent.

Call the Doctor

If you experience any of the following signs, contact your practitioner right away. Don't panic. Everything might be perfectly fine, but don't hesitate to make the call.

- Vaginal bleeding
- Abdominal cramping
- A severe headache
- Leaking something watery (amniotic fluid?)
- Painful and frequent urination
- Swollen joints, hands, or face
- Vomiting and nausea that is extreme, constant, and more than any morning sickness you may have experienced
- Dizziness or fainting
- A temperature higher than 101 degrees Fahrenheit

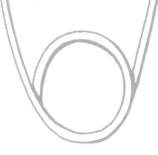

If Someone Uses the Expression . . .

- *Threatened miscarriage.* Your bleeding is light. You may even spot on and off for several days. Your cervix remains closed. You don't have great pain and losing your baby is not inevitable. Ultrasound will determine what's actually happening and a blood test will check the levels of HCG, the pregnancy hormone. A physical examination will not alter the circumstances one way or the other, but you will want to have a doctor's medical opinion and recommendations.

- *Inevitable miscarriage.* Your bleeding continues steadily. You have started to experience contractions. You may have low back pain or abdominal cramps. Your physician has discovered that your cervix is dilated. In this situation, a miscarriage is inevitable and will probably occur within twenty-four hours. If you notice that you are passing clots of blood, mixed with other fluids and you are in pain, you are in the midst of what is sometimes called a *spontaneous abortion.* In a complete and spontaneous miscarriage, all the placental and fetal tissue is expelled from your uterus. Sometimes a doctor may ask you to save the fetus and placenta in a clean container so it can be examined later. This may be simply impossible or emotionally tricky. However, keep in mind that your doctor is not trying to put you up to some horribly cruel task. His or her goal is to uncover what went wrong so it won't happen again. If your miscarriage is complete, your pain as well as the bleeding will stop and you'll be physically fine in a few days. Your uterus will even contract back to its prepregnant size.

- *Incomplete abortion.* Your body has expelled most of the placenta and fetus but not all. If parts remain in the uterus, you could experience heavy bleeding and your uterus will not be able to contract to stop the flow. Hemorrhaging is a possibility. A procedure called a *dilatation and curettage,* known simply as a "D & C" will be on your doctor's list of orders. During a D & C, your cervix is widened and the remaining tissue is scraped or suctioned out.

- *Missed abortion.* Occasionally, the fetus dies even earlier, in the first eight weeks of development, but remains in your womb. You don't experience any bleeding or pain, but you start to suspect something is not quite right. For instance, your breasts may not be quite as tender as they were earlier in your pregnancy. Or morning sickness could have disappeared. What's happened is that levels of HCG have dropped even though the fetus and placenta remain in your uterus. An ultrasound can confirm, and you will definitely be scheduled for a D & C. The diagnosis of a missed abortion used to be more common, but nowadays, close monitoring during this first trimester makes it less likely to miss for very long. Keep a record of your symptoms and if you suddenly "don't feel pregnant anymore," tell your doctor right away. Don't wait until your next appointment.

Why Do Miscarriages Occur?

About half the time, miscarriages are caused by chromosomal abnormalities in the fetus, or what's known as a blighted ovum. A random mistake of nature, a blighted ovum is not something you need to worry about in your future pregnancies.

Other factors to be considered in a miscarriage are:

- Hormonal deficiencies
- Anatomical problems in your cervix or uterus
- Incompatible blood types or the Rh factor
- Viruses and infections
- Immune disorders

The wave of emotions following a miscarriage run the gamut from grief, guilt, fear, anger, blame, frustration, and a real sense of personal failure. Others may not understand your feelings because your pregnancy may have been a very private affair up until this point. Yet, even though you may have been pregnant for only a few weeks, don't take this brief state of affairs lightly. Your dreams may have been dashed. The picture you created in your mind's eye of a happy baby was quite real—and so is your loss. Trying to pretend that it was no big deal is not the answer. Don't play the "If only"

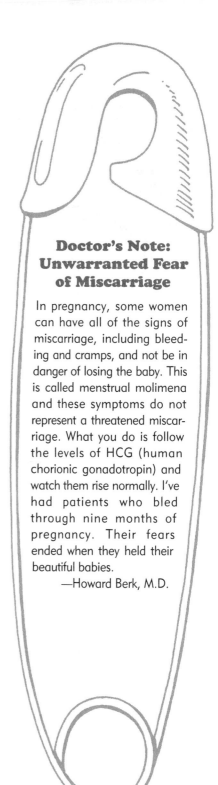

Doctor's Note: Unwarranted Fear of Miscarriage

In pregnancy, some women can have all of the signs of miscarriage, including bleeding and cramps, and not be in danger of losing the baby. This is called menstrual molimena and these symptoms do not represent a threatened miscarriage. What you do is follow the levels of HCG (human chorionic gonadotropin) and watch them rise normally. I've had patients who bled through nine months of pregnancy. Their fears ended when they held their beautiful babies.

—Howard Berk, M.D.

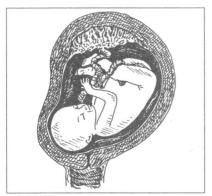

By the end of the third month, your fetus should show a completely human form.

game, either, thinking of endless "If only I hadn't carried groceries . . . had sex . . . exercised that morning . . . stayed up late . . . skipped my vitamins. . . . " Every woman is different and even a sense of relief can make you feel embarrassed or upset. You have a right to your emotions; and following a miscarriage, you can expect those emotions to swing wildly. Ask your doctor or someone at the hospital where you were going to deliver to recommend a counseling center or a group where you can share your grief.

Repeated miscarriage? It's important to speak with your doctor, who may want to schedule testing for genetic factors. Scar tissue, endometriosis, cysts, fibroid tumors, or damaged fallopian tubes can also be involved in miscarriages.

When Can I Get Pregnant Again?

Some doctors recommend that you wait at least three menstrual cycles before trying to become pregnant after a miscarriage. Others say it is quite safe to try right away. Every woman is different, and so are you. Don't go on hearsay. Go ahead and speak with your own practitioner, especially if you feel up to trying again right away.

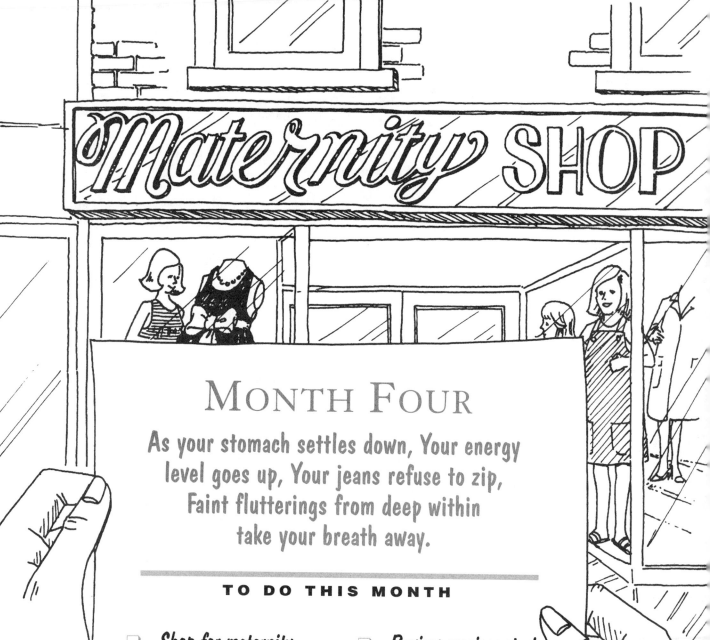

MONTH FOUR

As your stomach settles down, Your energy
level goes up, Your jeans refuse to zip,
Faint flutterings from deep within
take your breath away.

TO DO THIS MONTH

- ☐ *Shop for maternity clothes.*
- ☐ *Get ready to feel your unborn baby move.*
- ☐ *Go out for dinner.*
- ☐ *Review amniocentesis with your practitioner.*
- ☐ *Write down your dreams.*
- ☐ *Stay cool.*
- ☐ *Take your vitamins.*

It might be a Monday morning. Or a Friday. Perhaps it will hit you on a Saturday. You will wake up, slip to the edge of your bed, put your feet on the floor, and suddenly this state of pregnancy may strike you as something even more dramatic and earth-shattering than it has up until now. Yes, of course, on an intellectual, emotional, and certainly physical level, you've been growing into your expectant state for weeks and weeks. You are entering your fourth month, after all. However, on this particular morning, there's something else about your body that tells you: Yes, you are pregnant!

Your favorite outfits don't fit. Those jeans. That black suit. Your all-time, go-everywhere slacks and shirt. Your tried-and-true shorts for weekend gardening chores. Even your comfortable T-shirts are not quite what they used to be because they just don't fit right.

What Are You Feeling Emotionally?

At the Center for the Study of the Psychology of Pregnancy in California, director Nancy L. Robbins, MSW, once remarked, "Pregnancy is a great watershed—a profound life transition, after which nothing is ever the same again. During pregnancy, each woman looks deep within herself. It's a time of reevaluation and resolution—reevaluation of how you feel about yourself, your marriage, the relationship with your own parents and how you were raised. It reawakens years of unfinished business. The thoughtful inner work that must go on during this transition to motherhood is vital for each woman as she grows into her new role as mother."

What does all this have to do with your clothes not fitting anymore? A bit. In fact, perhaps more than just a bit. "When things go well," Robbins continued, "this inner turmoil results in feelings of confidence, independence, self-esteem. You come away from the crisis strengthened and adult. You experience the birth as a time of joy." In other words, you are not being frivolous or silly when you take your emotional state seriously. If you find yourself anxious, upset, frustrated, or struggling with a case of the "uglies," then go treat yourself to something beautiful today. Stay one step ahead of the physical changes of pregnancy, if you can, and you'll feel better emotionally.

Out of the mouths of other moms:

- "I would get depressed about getting dressed. Yet, I knew it was important for me to stay on an even keel emotionally. I stopped trying to squeeze into the old favorites in my closet and put them out of my sight."
- "I was getting up in the morning and trying on ten different outfits before I found one that snapped, buttoned, or didn't fit skintight."
- "It's so important to put yourself together neatly when you are pregnant. I know I am spending more time coordinating clothes and thinking about earrings, stockings, matching over-blouses to my regular turtlenecks and reassessing my final look, but it's worth it. My dad recently mentioned that I reminded him of my mother when she was pregnant. 'You look so neat,' he said, and I loved it."
- "Even though something might look ridiculous on a hanger, try it on. This is one stage of your life when you can't trust those old clothing instincts you thought you had narrowed down. Seriously, who would have ever thought I would be seen in a long, to-the-knee sweater and matching leg warmers."
- "Your own pregnancy shape is always a surprise when you spot yourself in a mirror or store window. For some reason, I guess because it comes on slowly month by month, you can't easily adjust to that big belly when you look at it squarely. Inside you are still your old body shape."

Let's Get Physical

During these middle three months of pregnancy, your second trimester, your growing belly becomes more obvious and, yes, getting dressed turns into a new adventure. On the positive side, you are feeling better and more energetic, and every day will become easier. Take a look at yourself in the mirror when you step out of the shower. Go ahead. Don't be afraid. That gentle rounding of your stomach is your baby. When your uterus is one finger's length below your navel, says obstetrician Howard Shapiro, you are approximately eighteen weeks pregnant.

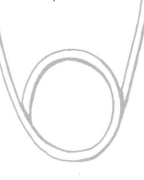

Soooo . . . Other Pregnant Women Have These Symptoms, Too:

- Tender breasts
- Fatigue
- Occasional dizziness
- Frequent urination
- Constipation
- Stomach as well as intestinal gas
- Bleeding gums
- Runny nose, stuffy sinuses
- Headaches
- Vaginal discharge
- Signs of varicose veins
- Feeling stuffed
- Weird changes in skin and hair
- Mildly swollen feet, ankles, face, or hands
- Flutters and burbling sensations from deep inside your womb

Funny Feelings and Flutterings?

Have you felt that faint fluttering that makes you think of tiny bubbles being blown inside or wings fluttering? Known as *quickening*, this marvelous sensation is your unborn child's growing life. Your practitioner may tell you that this indication of fetal movement is a wonderful way to determine how far along you are. If you are average, you'll detect these kicks, turns, flips, and pushes somewhere between the eighteenth and twentieth week. However, women who have already given birth can sense their baby's activity inside the womb as early as week 16 or 17 sometimes. According to spiritualists and some religious traditions, quickening sets the real beginning of a living human being.

In a Heartbeat

During your regular check-up this month, make sure that you and your partner take time to listen to the heartbeat.

Whew . . . Milestones & Side Effects

Not as Sick to Your Stomach

If you've been experiencing morning sickness, the nausea may ease up and disappear entirely.

Not as Sleepy

Your energy level should start to pick up. That inability to keep your eyes open because of overwhelming fatigue should taper off. So long sleepy-headedness.

Hungrier

Your appetite will increase and you can expect to gain from eleven to fifteen pounds, or 60 percent of your total maternity weight, in this trimester. Don't be a slave to that scale, however.

Amazed and Dazed by the Bodily Changes

Your nipples and the surrounding skin on your breasts may get darker in color. Meanwhile, a line running down the center of your stomach, called the *linea nigra*, might appear. Moles and freckles become more defined and darker. Don't worry. This isn't a sign of cancer. It just reflects an increase in skin pigmentation. You're quite normal.

Uh Oh . . . An Itchy and Uncomfortably Painful Backside

You could develop *hemorrhoids*, which are swollen rectal veins around your anus. These itchy, sore, possibly painful bloody vessels can be a real trial, especially when you try to go to the bathroom. If you haven't already discussed your problem with the doctor, do it now. Don't be shy. In the meantime, sit down. Standing or shopping for hours at a time can put unnecessary pressure on your veins there. In fact, sit on an ice pack. Ask for a prescription for a cream. Most mild cases of hemorrhoids do go away after delivery. By straining to have a bowel movement, you put stress on the rectal veins, which can become blocked, trapping blood, turning itchy, painful, and perhaps even protruding from the anus. Near the end of your nine months of pregnancy, the pressure of the baby can also add to this condition.

Bleeding or painful hemorrhoids should always be brought to your doctor's attention right away. You may have developed a blood clot. In the meantime, here are a few other things you can do:

- Dab a little petroleum jelly just inside your rectum before going to the bathroom.
- Climb into a tub filled with warm water and soak your backside, especially if your hemorrhoids are protruding. To shrink them, sit on an ice bag or a washcloth soaked in ice water as soon as you get out of the bathtub.
- Medicated wipes called Tucks can be a godsend. Keep them right next to your toilet. Your obstetrician may also prescribe a suppository kit.

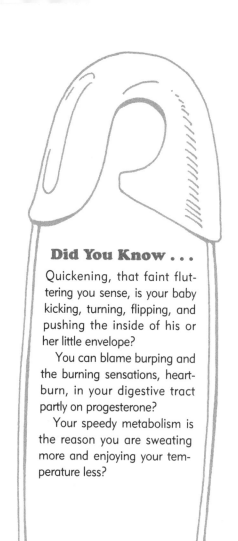

Did You Know . . .

Quickening, that faint fluttering you sense, is your baby kicking, turning, flipping, and pushing the inside of his or her little envelope?

You can blame burping and the burning sensations, heartburn, in your digestive tract partly on progesterone?

Your speedy metabolism is the reason you are sweating more and enjoying your temperature less?

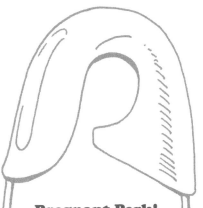

Pregnant Perk!

Insist on Help with Chores
Learn how to delegate without guilt. By doing everything yourself, you simply create dependency in the people around you. Dependency always turns into hostility sooner or later. Ask others to pitch in. When you feel pressed about a chore, think: what's the worst thing that will happen if I don't do this project? In many cases, not much. No one else may even notice.

- To relieve constipation, try eating plenty of high-fiber foods and drinking more water. Exercise regularly and take your prenatal vitamins on a full stomach with plenty of water. The extra iron in some manufacturer's brands can be compounding the problem in your bowels. Don't take over-the-counter laxatives, however, and do speak with your practitioner.

Breathless?

When you have sighing respirations and think, "Oh my God," it is not because you are breathless. The reason you feel this way is that you have to increase your vital capacity when you are pregnant. Your oxygen requirements are higher and, as a result, you lose certain reflexes that make a non-pregnant woman breathe without concern. Most people breathe and never even think about it. When you are pregnant, this changes and the inability to breathe freely without thinking can happen even when you aren't even moving. Don't panic. Stay calm for a few minutes and the sensation will go away. Meanwhile, pathological breathing is panting or breathing so rapidly that you start to feel faint. You can make yourself crazy, or become pathological, and actually pass out. However, fainting is a method of protecting your body. After you faint, or lose consciousness, you'll start breathing easier. When breathlessness is caused by anemia, it's rapid breathing after some kind of exertion.

Blood on Your Toothbrush

Your gums can become extrasensitive and may actually bleed when you brush your teeth. Take it easy. Make an appointment with your dentist to have your teeth cleaned, but be sure to tell him or her that you are pregnant. If you need to have X-rays taken, make sure the dentist or technician covers your abdomen with a lead shield.

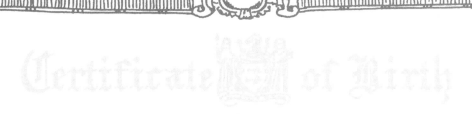

Warning Signs:
GET HELP

Severe Breathlessness: Diabetes, heart or blood disorders as well as a condition called hydroamnios, caused by too much amniotic fluid in the sac surrounding the fetus, can make it extremely difficult for you to catch your breath.

Vaginal Bleeding: Many women spot or bleed slightly in the first months. However, bleeding can be a sign of miscarriage or problems with the placenta.

Unusual thirst: Diabetes.

Severe swelling of the face or fingers: High blood pressure.

Blurry vision: High blood pressure.

Continuous or severe headache: Though this could be caused by anything from a sinus condition to an allergic response, headaches could also indicate that your body is retaining an excessive amount of fluid and toxemia, a very dangerous condition, is developing.

Severe abdominal pain: Miscarriage, premature labor, or problems with the placenta.

Fever or chills: You may have an infection.

Fluid discharge from your vagina: A sudden gush early in the first or second trimester could mean that you are leaking amniotic fluid. Such a leak could also mean that the amniotic sac has ruptured completely and labor could begin prematurely.

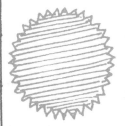

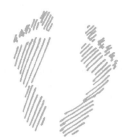

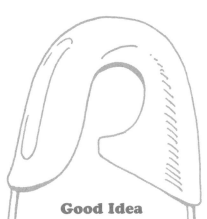

Good Idea

Stick with cotton underwear and aim for loose clothing. Tight-fitting exercise outfits or spandex tights can make your vaginal area sore. Speak with your doctor about his recommendations for making you feel better. Deodorant soaps, perfumes, and bubble baths will undoubtedly be on a list of no-no's for now. Don't even attempt to douche unless you get full instructions ahead of time. Douching, in some cases, can be dangerous for your unborn baby. If the discharge appears to be yellow, green, smells like a loaf of bread, or has a foul odor, you may have *vaginitis*, an infection. You may also be aware of a burning, itching, or sore vagina if this is the case. An ointment or cream should be able to help. Get good advice and a prescription, however.

Sticky Discharge on Your Underpants

Have you noticed an increase in a thin, sticky, white discharge, similar to the kind you may have experienced just before your monthly period? If so, you've got a normal situation known as *leukorrhea* and not necessarily vaginitis, an infection. For some women, the leukorrhea increases to a point where they decide to wear a sanitary pad. Don't reach for a tampon, however. You don't want to risk introducing any germs into your vagina when you are pregnant. The discharge is really nothing to worry about even if it makes you feel uncomfortable. If you develop more annoying symptoms, such as pain, itching, redness, or swelling and a change in discharge consistency as well as color, call your doctor.

Vaginal Infections

Even if you haven't been one of those women prone to vaginitis (infections of the vagina), now that you are pregnant, some experts say that you are ten times more likely to develop one. Rest assured that simple vaginitis is not going to harm your baby. There are actually three types of vaginitis, according to obstetrician Harold Shapiro: trichomoniasis, moniliasis, and bacterial vaginosis. *Moniliasis*, or yeast infection, may be the most common one for expectant moms. You may also have a fungus called *Candida albicans* in your vagina. An overgrowth of this fungus will give you a case of cottage cheesy discharge, itching vulva, and red and swollen vagina. Let's face it, everything about your biochemistry is thrown off by the pregnancy, so why should the climate in your vagina be any different. Because there is concern about the unborn baby contracting the infection during the birth, you'll want to clear it up as soon as possible:

- Talk to your doctor and get tested. You need to rule out any sexually transmitted infections. A sample of your secretion may be needed to get the full story.
- Use an ice pack to soothe the itching. Applications of witch hazel may also relieve some of your frustrating and itchy symptoms.
- Boric acid capsules and ointments may be recommended.
- Eating yogurt, which contains lactobacilus-acidophilus or the active cultures, could help. What you want to do is restore the

right bacterial balance in your vagina and the yogurt actually has some of the very same organisms your body may need.

- Stay as clean and as dry as you can.
- Wear cotton underpants and avoid tight-fitting pants.

Icch . . . Heartburn!

First of all, you need to know that heartburn has nothing to do with your heart. If you've been experiencing a burning sensation in your throat and chest, the cause is indigestion. The acid in your stomach is backing up into your esophagus. Your growing uterus isn't helping matters either as it grows and begins to push up on your stomach. Countless pregnant women have moaned and groaned their way through nine months of burping and burning gastrointestinal upset. Hormones relax all your smooth muscle tissue, even the ones in your digestive tract. Food moves more slowly through your system. In fact, some people say that the slower it goes, the better off your baby may be because you are getting a lot more nutrient absorption.

Oh What a Relief It Is . . . Help for Heartburn:

- Skip the greasy fries.
- Cut down on fatty foods.
- Try many small meals, instead of three square ones a day.
- Drink lots of water. Although they may be sending you to the bathroom more than you like, fluids can help reduce that buildup of acid in your stomach.
- Don't eat just before you go to bed or are about to lie down to rest.
- Shop for loose-fitting maternity clothes. Squeezing into your old jeans puts pressure on your stomach area.
- Try an antacid such as Mylanta, Maalox, Riopan, Milk of Magnesia. Tablets that could ease your upset are Gelusil, Rolaids, or Tums.
- Tums is the best antacid for pregnancy because it also supplies you with the extra calcium you need. Take two Tums after each meal and two before going to bed for a week. If you have also eliminated fried foods, your heartburn should be

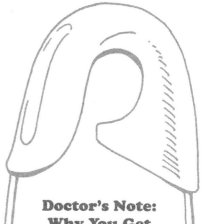

Doctor's Note: Why You Get Heartburn

The progesterone that your body manufactures during pregnancy produces a relaxation of the connection between the esophagus and the stomach for a very good reason. As you get further along in pregnancy, your stomach may not be able to distend because the uterus is in the way. Therefore, you need an escape valve. When there is no room for your food to move down, the relaxed connection makes it easier to come back up. The result for you is heartburn.

—Howard Berk, M.D.

EVERYTHING PREGNANCY BOOK

gone. If it's not, then you have to consult with your physician because your heartburn may not be a simple thing. You can actually end up with gastrointestinal bleeding from heartburn. "I have my patients use drugs like Pepcid and Zantac," says Dr. Berk. Work with your doctor to find the right medicine.

- Raising the head of your bed when you sleep or nap can help. Put six inch blocks or even a couple of sturdy books under the mattress. Adding a pillow or two simply won't be as effective.
- Stay away from alcohol, cola, tea, coffee, chocolate, peppermint, and spearmint: these may relax the valve between the stomach and the esophagus, according to Richard Berkowitz, M.D., and Rosemary Wein, RN, of Mount Sinai. This relaxation lets the contents of your stomach back up.
- Write down what you eat for a couple of days. You may be able to figure out which foods are the worst offenders. Although highly spicy meals, tomatoes, and citrus fruits or juices are known culprits, your own body may be reacting to another food group entirely.

Oh Baby . . . Inside Secrets Now

Fetal growth is quite dramatic and rapid now. Sleeping and waking, moving, sucking, swallowing, and passing urine, the fetus looks more like a miniature human being every day. While the head has been disproportionately large up until this point, the body is now catching up in size:

- Length stretches from four to eight or ten inches, which could be up to nearly half of what it will be at birth.
- Weight shoots up from one to six ounces.
- Facial features are distinct with eyebrows and eyelashes.
- Thin, nearly transparent skin is covered with a fine, downy hair known as *lanugo*. Blood vessels beneath the skin are visible.
- Thumb-suckers show their penchants to put hand to mouth.
- Bone shapes are growing and signs of the skeleton can be seen. From what are known as ossification centers will come

the bone cells that fill in and harden. However, this growth process is one that continues long after birth and well into adolescence and young adulthood.

- Breathing movements can be seen as the fetus's chest moves in and out. During this fourth month, the heart is pumping blood strong enough and loud enough for you and your doctor to hear.

- Fetal blood is being pumped through this little body at about four miles an hour. Instead of going to the developing lungs to obtain fresh oxygen and get rid of carbon dioxide, the fetal blood is pushed out through two large arteries in the umbilical cord and on to the placenta, which looks like a dish, is about three inches in diameter now, and has a unique network of blood vessels. On the way back to the fetus, the blood travels through one large umbilical vein. According to obstetrician and researcher Virginia Apgar, this round trip of fetal blood—through the cord, to the placenta, and back to the tiny little body—takes only about thirty seconds.

- Your placenta is actually a multidimensional organ that takes care of the work of the lungs, kidneys, intestines, liver, and hormone-producing parts of the fetus's life. There are two sides to the placenta: a maternal and a fetal. The placenta's marvelous biochemistry makes it possible for nutrients to pass and wastes to be removed. Your unborn baby's waste products, urine and carbon dioxide, are picked up in the placenta and eventually excreted through your own kidneys and lungs.

- The umbilical cord is about as long as the fetus and continues to grow. The average umbilical cord at birth is up to twenty-four inches, but it can be as short as five inches and as long as forty-eight inches. Pressure from the blood being continually pumped through it helps straighten the cord out and keeps it from becoming knotted or getting in the way of your unborn baby's kicks and somersaults.

- Sex organs are now visible, although ultrasound scans can still miss this bit of information at times.

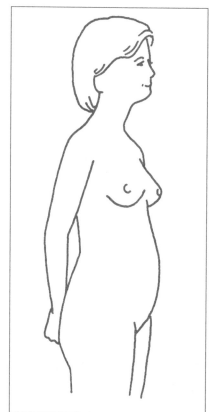

At the beginning of the second trimester, your stomach will show a gentle rounding, and you will start to lose your waistline.

Certificate of Birth

Placenta Pride!

"In many ways, the placenta is the SCUBA system for the fetus while at the same time being the Houston Control Center guiding the mother through pregnancy," explains Harvey J. Kliman, Ph.D., from the Department of Obstetrics and Gynecology at Yale University School of Medicine. "The placenta is dedicated to the survival of the fetus. Even when exposed to a poor maternal environment—malnourishment, disease, cigarette smoking, or cocaine—the placenta can often compensate by becoming more efficient." Don't push your luck, however. As Dr. Kliman says, "Unfortunately, there are limits to the placenta's ability to cope with external stresses."

Trained placenta pathologists can actually see what happened during a pregnancy by examining placental tissue, especially in cases where something went wrong and parents are anxious to know the hard facts. "Just as the rings of a cut tree can tell the story of a tree's life," Kliman says, "so too can the placenta disclose the history of a pregnancy. In cases of poor outcome, microscopic examination reveals the stresses that caused fetal damage in the newborn."

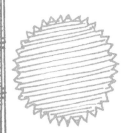

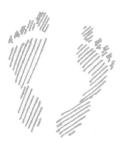

In Your Doctor's Bag of Tools and Tests

You may be scheduled for an alpha-fetoprotein (AFP) test.

Your unborn baby is producing a protein, known as AFP, and passing it into your circulatory system. This screening blood test, performed by simply drawing blood, to check the level of AFP may be done to find out if you are carrying twins. Most of the time, a high level of AFP accounts for more than one baby. However, it could mean that your fetus has a neural tube defect. So, if you have a high level, you should have a sonogram to check for the presence of more than one baby. With low AFP, amniocentesis is definitely indicated. The AFP, done between the sixteenth and eighteenth weeks, can also indicate the possibility of Down's syndrome or neural tube defects, which occur once in every 1,000 births. If you have already had a baby with anencephaly or spina bifida, your chances of having another child with a neural tube defect increase significantly. Results of the AFP test are usually available within one week, but the reliability of the outcome is imprecise if your due date hasn't been accurately calculated, if you have diabetes, or you are carrying twins. If the AFP levels are high, the practitioner may recommend a second test or request that you have an ultrasound right away. Rest assured that only a small number of women who have irregular AFP test results actually do give birth to babies with birth defects, according to the American College of Obstetricians and Gynecologists.

An AFP-3 test is a bit more sophisticated than the simple AFP test, but it has proven to pick up signs of Down's syndrome. In what is called a triple screen test, the technician measures your AFP as well as the level of human chorionic gonadotropin (HCG) and estriol, a type of estrogen, in your blood. High HCG and low estriol are signs of possible danger.

A Doctor's Note: Let's Get Specific

There is now a test called the Quad test that checks AFP, chorionic gonadotropin, estriol, and inhibin. This new diagnostic tool will probably help to decrease the number of amniocentesis performed because it is so specific. Whenever a medical test is designed, you have to make sure it suits patients at either end of the spectrum. When a test isn't as specific as it could be, you end up with lots of false or confusing results. Patients are told that the test was negative when the news is actually positive. With this new Quad test, practitioners are going to be able to restrict the number of misleading readings. Remember, all of this testing is only a screening procedure, which may indicate that further study is necessary. Amniocentesis and ultrasound will give the final answer.

—Howard Berk, M.D.

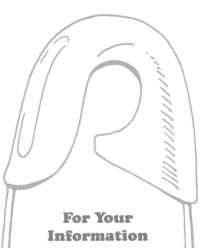

**For Your
Information**

During conception, when your mate's sperm and your egg unite, each brings twenty-three chromosomes. In a case of Down's syndrome, an extra chromosome is contributed. This one is called *Trisomy 21* (*trisomy*, three chromosomes) and can be detected in the results of amniocentesis. A baby with Downs syndrome will be born with very distinct features, including slanting, closely set eyes, a thick tongue, short neck, as well as abnormal hands and feet. Short in stature throughout life and mentally retarded, Down's syndrome children have been making great intellectual strides in recent years. Some also have congenital heart disease or respiratory problems.

You may be a candidate for amniocentesis.

The water, or amniotic fluid, inside the sac where your unborn baby is growing, can offer experts incredibly detailed information about the developing new life inside you. *Amniocentesis* is the procedure that makes this screening possible. Under ultrasound guidance, to avoid touching your unborn baby, a needle is inserted into the amniotic sac and amniotic fluid is drawn. Fetal cells are pulled from the fluid and are grown in a laboratory culture for chromosomal analysis. Long before birth, your unborn baby's new life is examined. Not only can the age and sex be determined, but also genetic disorders, metabolic problems, and other kinds of birth defects can be discovered.

Amniocentesis is performed sometime between the fourteenth and eighteenth week of pregnancy. Since you are in your fourth month, this may be an issue you are now facing. Here are reasons why an amniocentesis may be planned during this second trimester:

- Are you over thirty-five? Almost all obstetricians in the United States will recommend that you have one if you are over 35 because the risk of carrying a baby with Down's syndrome starts to rise as you get older. However, some doctors believe that using the age of thirty-five is a bit arbitrary. If you are in your thirties and this is your first pregnancy and you are concerned, you may want to schedule the test anyway. When the father is over fifty, amniocentesis could be advised because there may be a connection between paternal age and an increased risk of Down's syndrome.
- Have you had a baby with a genetic disorder? If you've already had a baby with a hereditary or chromosomal abnormality, an amniocentesis could make you feel more comfortable.
- Is their a concern about infection?
- Has your Rh status come up?
- Is there any history of neural tube defects (spina bifida), hemophilia, Tay-Sachs disease, or sickle-cell anemia in your family?
- Were your AFP test results worrisome? Even if there is no medical history of concern, if alpha-fetoprotein (AFP), a substance that is produced by the baby in the womb and that passes into your bloodstream, shows up at a higher than normal level, an amnio may help clear up any questions.

Amniocentesis sounds a bit scary . . .
How is the test performed?

Ouch, you may be saying. The very idea of someone puncturing your womb with a needle sounds unpleasant. Yet, discomfort may be minimal and the reason for having an amniocentesis could be important. Thousands and thousands of amniocentesis tests are performed routinely without complications. Only 1 in every 100 women experience complications, such as cramps or even a miscarriage (1 in 200 women). You may even be able to have the test done right there in the doctor's office. At the very most, you'll have to go to the hospital or clinic as an outpatient. Most centers insist on a visit to a genetic counselor who will discuss risks before you sign a consent form. Amniocentesis usually takes only a few minutes, thirty at the most, from beginning to end. Make sure to take your husband or close friend along with you for moral support.

Once you are up on the examining table, the technician will clean the bare skin on your abdomen with an antiseptic solution. The goal of this test is to obtain a vial of your amniotic fluid using a needle that will penetrate right through to the sac that protects your baby. Yes, it may hurt.

Local anesthetic applied to the site at which the needle will be injected can actually feel worse than amniocentesis. Discuss ways of dealing with your discomfort with both your doctor and the technician. Some experts have found that deep relaxation exercises, as well as hypnotism, can make the test go smoother.

One of the reasons for waiting until the fourteenth or fifteenth week is that there is more amniotic fluid present and the likelihood of sticking the fetus, the placenta, or the umbilical cord with a misplaced needle is low. However, the primary reason to wait until this point in pregnancy is that your fetus will have more cells being sloughed off. Earlier, there may be very few cells present in the amniotic fluid. The results of the test might indicate that everything is fine when, in fact, there weren't enough cells for a true test.

If someone suggests that you have an amniocentesis before the fifteenth week, ask about having a specialist handle the technique. Needle injuries are very rare because the technician's aim is

Exactly, What Is a Neural Tube Defect?

When the nervous system in your fetus does not develop properly early in pregnancy, the unborn baby can develop what experts call a *neural tube defect*. Nervous tissue may not completely be covered by skin or scalp. The spinal cord can be affected. The baby's brain doesn't always grow adequately. Neural tube defects produce fetuses with abnormally large heads and or water on the brain. Spina bifida, or exposed nerve tissue at the base of the fetal spine, may mean that your baby will be paralyzed in the legs. The degree of this defect can vary. In some cases, the baby will die soon after birth while in others, the problem is minor.

guided by an ultrasound picture every step of the way. Even sudden somersaults or changes in fetal positioning are taken into consideration. Clear amniotic fluid is drawn up and then rapidly sent to the lab for evaluation. The technician will also watch your fetus for a few minutes on the ultrasound screen to make sure everything is fine. Your unborn baby's heart rate is checked. Afterward, you may have a few cramps or a bit of vaginal bleeding. Very slight leaks of amniotic fluid have also been noted. You won't have any restrictions on activity afterward if everything has gone fine.

Yes, There Are a Few Real Risks . . .

Understanding the possible complications of amniocentesis is important, but try not to dwell on disasters. The American College of Obstetricians and Gynecologists (ACOG) reports only 1 in 200 women will have a miscarriage as a result of amniocentesis. A very small minority have reported trauma to the unborn baby, bleeding in either the placenta or the umbilical cord, inadvertent rupture of the sac, amniotic fluid infections, premature labor, and spontaneous abortion. If you are unlucky enough to experience any aftereffects, call your doctor immediately. You may end up in bed for a few days, but chances are excellent that any leakage or bleeding will stop without further medical intervention. In cases where the needle has actually nicked the baby, doctors can usually see the mark on the skin at birth. Long-term follow-up studies of mothers and babies who have taken advantage of this test show no problems at all.

The worst thing about amniocentesis could be the timing. Because the lab needs up to two weeks to complete the evaluation of the fetal cells in the fluid, you could be forced to face some tough issues at this point in your pregnancy. Why so long for the test results? For a diagnosis, the small sample of fetal cells in the fluid must be grown in a culture. This can take weeks. If you fall into one of those high-risk categories and are waiting to decide whether to proceed with your pregnancy, you could be living on the razor's edge emotionally. By the time the test results are back, you will be halfway through your pregnancy, or close to being twenty weeks pregnant. Not only have you become emotionally attached to this unborn being, but second-trimester terminations are more difficult to perform and have a higher risk of complications.

When faced with an amniocentesis:

- Pull your calendar out (How far along will you be when you receive the news?).
- Consider all the issues (For instance, do you want to know the sex of your baby before birth or would you rather wait?).
- Discuss all your concerns with your practitioner before you schedule the test.

I Was Wondering . . .

My dreams have been so vivid and wild. Is this because I'm pregnant?

Vivid and emotionally powerful dreams are very typical during pregnancy and immediately after delivery. Although no medical studies can confirm the connection between your elevated hormone levels and your very active dream state, experts do say that there is a link. Let's face it, hormones have been proven to affect emotions. When you are pregnant, the level of estrogen and progesterone in your body is higher than ever, so why wouldn't the hormonal storm brew up a batch of wild dreams, fantasies, and fears. Not only is your chemistry having an impact on your nighttime imagination, but also the simple fact of facing such a life-altering event enters the picture. If you are waiting for results from an amniocentesis test, if you are unhappy with the way your body is changing, if your morning sickness has refused to disappear quietly, then the emotional and physical battles you fight during the day have a way of spilling over into the night.

If you clearly recall your dream upon awakening, analysts suggest that you try to figure out the emotion left behind. Are you happy? Sad? Scared? Calm? Angry? You might even want to write down anything you can recall from the dream. Put a pad and pen next to your bed and do this immediately because dreams have a way of slipping away. Read your notes back later. If you can identify the emotion, connect it to a feeling in your life. What is making you happy, sad, scared, calm, angry? If you are feeling happy or calm, there is no problem at all. However, if your dreams are closer to nightmares and you end up fearful, scared, sad, or angry, you may want to talk to your mate, your practitioner, a good friend, or a counselor. Dreaming in pregnancy could be a way for you to face your deep-seated emotional puzzles.

Why am I so hot and sweaty all the time?

Relax. You're normal. Your metabolism works overtime during pregnancy. Like an overheated engine, your body is burning more calories even when you are simply sitting still. An increase in blood supply to the surface of your skin and all the raging hormones in your pregnant biochemistry add to the heat and sweat, too. To look and feel better, plan ahead. Don't dress in polyester clothes. Choose loose layers of cotton, instead, so you can take off pieces as you start to perspire. Open windows at night to make sleeping more comfortable. Invest in a room air conditioner if you must. Your sleep and comfort are important during pregnancy. Tell your mate to put on a sweater if he's too cold. Hop in the shower to cool off. Try patting on a little talcum powder afterward. Investigate antiperspirants if your regular one isn't meeting your increased needs. Drink water to replace all the fluids you are losing through sweat. You don't want to become dehydrated.

Can pregnancy be causing my nasal congestion and allergy flare-ups?

Yes. For some women, pregnancy can feel like a bad head cold complete with stuffy nose, yucky mucus, congestion, and the kind of postnasal drip that makes you want to gag or choke. The high levels of estrogen and progesterone circulating and the increased volume of blood reaching all your mucus membranes can make the lining of your respiratory tract swell. You may even see nose bleeds as a result. Experts say that this annoying side effect is harmless and will go away after your baby is born. Unfortunately, if you've always had problems with hay fever, sneezing, itchy, and teary eyes during particular allergy seasons, you may be even worse off. Yet, women with no previous history of allergies can also find themselves in this itching, sneezing, nose-blowing situation.

Speak with your doctor about remedies because there are safe medications available. Ask about taking extra vitamin C. If you are pregnant in the winter and the dry air is wreaking havoc on the delicate, sore skin of your nostrils, use a humidifier. In the meantime, try not to blow your nose too violently.

If your nose does start to bleed, don't lie on your back or lean backward. Sit down, lean forward very slightly, and try blowing gently to remove any clot. If that doesn't work, stick a bit of wet cotton or sterile gauze in the bleeding nostril. Pinch your nose between your thumb and forefinger with the gauze or cotton in place. Let your packing stay put for a few minutes and don't tug it out forcefully. Lean over a sink and wet it again when you think the bleeding has stopped. You can also try putting an ice pack on your nose. The cold should shrink the blood vessels and reduce bleeding. Nasal cauterization could be indicated if you are having recurring, severe nosebleeds. The nasal mucus membranes respond like your uterus with dilatation of blood vessels. Therefore, if you have a large vessel that is continually bleeding, it may have to be cauterized by your practitioner.

Could I be losing my mind? I keep forgetting things and I've never been a scatter-brain?

No, you aren't going crazy. Like other pregnancy symptoms linked to the hormonal storm brewing in your body, your ability to remain clear-headed is being undermined. It's normal and not lifelong. Some experts liken your foggy feeling to the same sensations you may have had at particular times of your monthly menstrual cycle. Try making lists for your essential to-do's. Reduce the stress in your life, if possible. For instance, don't rush and don't expect more of yourself now than you would have been accomplishing every day even before you were pregnant. Stop aiming for 100 percent efficiency in everything you do.

I'm worried about getting enough calcium in my diet because I just don't like milk. How much should I be consuming?

You need 50 percent more calcium a day or at least 1,200 milligrams. Calcium is really important throughout pregnancy, but especially in the

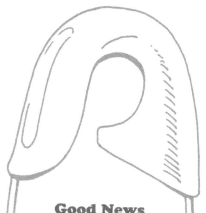

Good News

If you find yourself in a high-risk category, make sure that your doctor is up-to-date on all the latest advances in prenatal testing. The accuracy and safety of these screening techniques are changing constantly. In fact, in the latest breakthrough report, a new combination of blood tests is allowing experts to uncover genetic disorders, as well as Down's syndrome, before fifteen weeks of pregnancy. Having the information you need about your baby in the first trimester is so critical. The new tests look at another pregnancy-related protein, simply called A, as well as your HCG levels.

second and third trimesters, because your unborn baby is developing bone and blood cells. Some experts believe that in the second half of pregnancy, the unborn baby will use as much as thirteen milligrams of calcium per hour. The baby's nervous system, muscles, and teeth also depend on your calcium intake. Milk and dairy products are great sources, of course, but you can also get calcium from sardines, mackerel, salmon, broccoli, other green leafy vegetables like kale, collard, and turnip greens as well as calcium-enriched orange juice. Tums can add calcium and help fight heartburn, too. Experiment with sources of calcium. Ask your doctor about recommendations. Find a milk product you like. Are you a cheese lover? Or do you enjoy ice cream? To help your body absorb calcium, make sure that you are getting enough vitamin D, which speeds up the absorption of calcium. By making a habit of adding calcium to your diet now, you can head off the risk of developing osteoporosis later in life.

My sister has two cats and I was planning to visit her for a few days. Should I be worried about getting toxoplasmosis?

Your fear of *toxoplasmosis*, a virus that can affect your baby in the womb, is very legitimate. When cats are allowed to roam freely outside, eating anything and everything, especially wild animals or raw meat, they can end up with a parasite that settles in the intestines and is excreted into kitty litter boxes. You just don't want to catch this parasite. If you do, you may feel like you have a mild case of the flu for a few days and you'll quickly recover. The real danger is to your unborn baby, which has a 40 percent chance of being touched by the toxoplasmosis and being born blind, deaf, or mentally handicapped as a result. Keep in mind that toxoplasmosis in pregnancy is rare and that most house cats don't eat wild prey, but stick to canned goods as a rule. Are your sister's cats allowed to run outside? How long has she had them? If they are strictly house-bound, then you don't need to be as concerned. Don't offer to clean her kitty litter box no matter what kind of cats she has, however. Before you go, you can also ask your doctor to perform a blood test to determine if you've already had a case of toxoplasmosis, which would have resulted in your having antibodies in your blood. Speak with your doctor about your concerns.

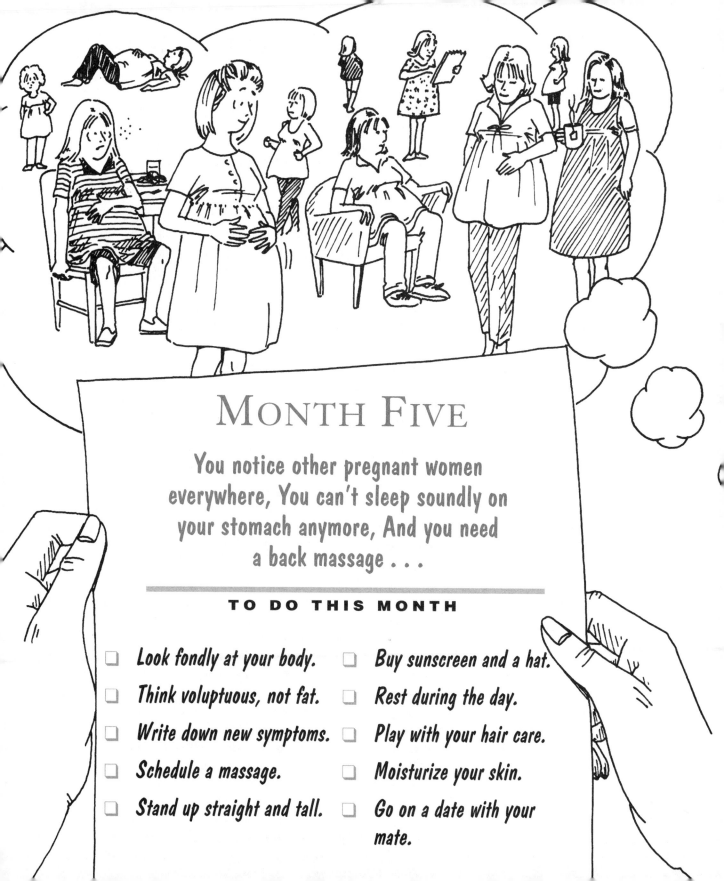

MONTH FIVE

You notice other pregnant women everywhere, You can't sleep soundly on your stomach anymore, And you need a back massage . . .

TO DO THIS MONTH

- ☐ *Look fondly at your body.*
- ☐ *Think voluptuous, not fat.*
- ☐ *Write down new symptoms.*
- ☐ *Schedule a massage.*
- ☐ *Stand up straight and tall.*
- ☐ *Buy sunscreen and a hat.*
- ☐ *Rest during the day.*
- ☐ *Play with your hair care.*
- ☐ *Moisturize your skin.*
- ☐ *Go on a date with your mate.*

I hate to admit it, but I have to be honest. I gained forty-five pounds during my first pregnancy and I thought I looked okay. A friend gained fourteen and felt fat.

All mothers look back on their pregnant bodies either with fondness, remembering the fun they had with the amusing shape they were in, or with misery, recalling only how awful they felt about themselves and how huge they believed they looked to the world. It doesn't seem quite fair, because the difference between the two pregnancies—one happy and one miserable—is not based on pounds but on attitude, according to some experts. While it is not possible to wish away any aches and pains of pregnancy, your state of mind can definitely affect the degree of your distress. A case of the emotional uglies will make you feel worse physically.

How Are You Feeling About Your Body?

Fat? The first step toward getting rid of your "fatty-fatty-two-by-four" attitude is to understand a few of the faulty errors of logic behind your feelings of inferiority. It's not always your fault when you dislike your pregnant body, and knowing where your attitude comes from could take you half the distance toward seeing yourself as voluptuous, not fat.

Error No. 1: The Medical Standard for a Perfect Pregnancy Weight Gain Is Reasonable

It's not. Although there has been a giant leap for womankind from twenty years ago, when women were tortured officially if they gained more than eighteen pounds, the American College of Obstetricians and Gynecologists (ACOG) still says that twenty to thirty pounds is ideal. Perhaps it is. Meanwhile, a majority of women gain more than thirty pounds, according to nurse-midwife Lonnie Morris, who has been directing the Childbirth Center in Englewood, New Jersey, for more than twenty years. "Gains of twenty-five to thirty-five pounds have the best outcomes in pregnancy," Morris says. It's only when a woman gains more than fifty pounds that there is a need for her to worry that she will lose her figure.

The ACOG ideal is not a standard every single average, healthy, pregnant woman can meet. This woman is set up to fail. And, determined to be thin again, she may diet herself into a dangerous preoccupation with her weight.

Error No. 2: All Your Pregnancy Weight Gain Should Be in the Stomach Area

Wrong. You need to gain weight all over when you are pregnant to keep your balance, among other reasons. Some of these additional pounds may settle in your lower torso—on all of those hot spots of emotional upset for women: thighs, hips, buttocks. My obstetrician once told me that if my entire pregnancy weight gain had been only in my stomach, I would have had a difficult time walking without falling forward.

Error No. 3: Many Maternity Clothes Manufacturers Still Assume Pregnancy Is Something to Hurry Through and Hide

It shouldn't be. Years ago, I spent some time researching maternity clothes for a special project. I talked to hundreds of people in the fashion and garment industry and often encountered the attitude—sometimes outspoken, sometimes only hinted at—that pregnancy isn't a very pretty time of life. Although some experts spoke of the special maternity glow an expectant woman is expected to have, it's an idea, they said, that often eludes women.

When I told one industry businessman that I was writing about maternity fashion, he replied, "Maternity and fashion are mutually exclusive terms. Pregnant women can't really be fashionable. They are fat and swollen." Can you believe that his philosophy has had no effect on his designers?

I saw labels for customers who wanted to "dress for success" and interviewed individuals who claimed to have new leases on pregnant life, but the clothes by many designers are still supposed to look good "in spite of" pregnancy, not because of it. Why is it a compliment to tell a woman expecting a baby "You don't even look pregnant!"?

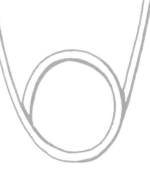

Soooo . . . Other Pregnant Women Have These Symptoms, Too:

- Tender breasts
- Fatigue
- Occasional dizziness
- Frequent urination
- Constipation
- Stomach as well as intestinal gas
- Bleeding gums
- Runny nose, stuffy sinuses
- Headaches
- Vaginal discharge
- Feeling stuffed
- Weird changes in skin and hair
- Mildly swollen feet, ankles, face, or hands
- Flutters and burbling sensations from deep inside your womb

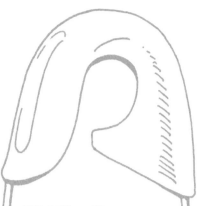

Error No. 4: "I Hate My Body, and Clothes Won't Help"

They will. When maternity clothes are churned out for mass marketing, cheap fabrics are used (no one will want to wear them very long, businesses insist); few variations in size are allowed (why have a garment cut and fit correctly when you are simply getting through?); and the rationale behind design is, how can we help a woman camouflage her unsightly shape? If a woman has a lot of money to spend or is particularly inventive, she can sidestep these cheap solutions. Many women, however, don't have the time, the money, or the inclination to invent their wardrobes when they are expecting. They end up looking in the mirror, not liking what they see—falsely assuming the problem is the body, not the clothes.

"What I've always hated about American maternity clothes is their childishness," one mother told me. "When I was pregnant, for the first time in my life I was really busty . . . and I wanted to show it off. But everything I saw was frilly and childish. It's such a contradiction. You are pregnant, and obviously you've had sex with someone, and there are suddenly all these manufacturers who are trying to dress you up as a little girl."

Error No. 5: You Should Look Like the Fashion Models in Maternity Ads

Wrong. Usually, they are not pregnant. One maternity catalog owner actually said that using women who are really pregnant to model her clothes is always a mistake. "Pregnant faces, legs, and arms look fat when photographed," she explained to my horror. Then, she mentioned that a better option was to rely upon a company that makes fake pregnancy pillows. Ouch. Therefore, too often, when a pregnant woman admires a dress in an ad and imagines resembling the model, she's picturing herself unpregnant . . . with a pillow strapped to her stomach. There's a big, unfair difference between the two.

Did You Know . . .

All of your weight gain won't be in your stomach area. It's normal to be putting on pounds in other places—hips, thighs, buttocks, and arms, too?

Vernix is the white, greasy, protective substance that now covers your unborn baby's little body in his watery world?

The top of your uterus is up to your belly button?

Normally, you lose 100 hairs a day. During pregnancy, there is no fallout so it's thicker?

Oh Baby . . . Inside Secrets Now

- Your unborn baby may grow two more inches this month, which will bring length anywhere from ten inches up to fourteen or fifteen.
- Weight will move from six ounces, up to a full pound by month's end.
- Your unborn baby is growing hair on his or her head.
- Teeth are developing and minuscule tooth buds for permanent teeth are already there, too.
- Skin is still see-through, so the fetal blood vessels appear to glow. Silvery little bones are visible but starting to harden in this second trimester.
- A white greasy substance called *vernix* will soon protect the skin in its watery, womb environment. Secreted by tiny glands in the skin, sebum, an oily film first appears before becoming waxy and thick to form the vernix. Like any marathon swimmer getting ready for a long-distance race, your unborn baby needs this greasy protection. My son Zach, who was born two weeks before his official delivery date, came into the world still wearing a complete outfit of vernix. On his first glimpse of Zach, my husband announced that his son was born with a coating of cheesecake.
- Arms and legs are well formed and are still covered by the soft, silky hair known as lanugo. Most of this fetal hair is rubbed off and disappears before birth.
- The unborn baby can grip firmly with hands now.
- Noises from the outside world are noticed. The fetus recognizes your voice and has actually been shown to startle at the sound of loud crashes or bangs. The sounds of your digestive tract and your heartbeat are heard clearly inside.
- Fluttering, kicking, somersaulting, twisting, and turning, the unborn baby may be most active at predictable times. Rest and sleep are also on the daily fetal must-do list. In fact, some unborn babies have been known to respond to the rocking and gentle motions of their mothers long before they

Your Uterus? A Two-Part Harmony

There are two main parts of your uterus, the primary organ of pregnancy:

1. The upper, or *corpus*, is muscular and can expand. Its top is sometimes referred to as the fundus.
2. The uterine mouth or the cervix. During these last three months and most dramatically in labor and delivery, these two parts work together contracting and pushing the baby down until the cervix dilates (opens).

see the light of real day. This may explain why your baby sleeps more when you are active during the day. In the evening, with your feet up, finally relaxed in your favorite chair or propped up on the bed with a pile of pillows for comfort, you can't quite drift off or give in to your fatigue because it's exercise time in the womb! Have your mate stick around to see and feel the action.

Let's Get Physical

The top of your uterus has reached your navel by now. Put your finger there to see if you can feel it. Meanwhile, some of the same problems that plagued you last month may refuse to disappear.

Consider Yourself Normal If . . .

- You have begun to experience occasional twinges of pain or dull aches in your lower abdomen. Common between the eighteenth and twenty-fourth weeks of pregnancy, these simply mean that your uterus is growing and the ligaments that support it on either side are being pulled and stretched. Don't turn quickly from your waist. Change your position if you sit for long periods. When you feel a tug, bend into where the pain is originating. Don't forget to tell your practitioner.
- Your back aches. As your weight distribution changes, so does the way you stand, sit, walk, and move. All this can put strain on your back muscles and an achy back can begin somewhere in mid-pregnancy and continue right on up to delivery day and beyond. What may also begin to bother you during this fifth month is a condition called *lumbar lordosis*. Your lower spine is curving forward. Common and terribly annoying, the pain is caused by your spine twisting itself to make space for the baby inside. A substance called *relaxin* is circulating in your body and the more relaxin, the more curved your spine becomes. Your muscles, meanwhile, aren't always happy about this shift

and they let you know when they ache. Half of all pregnant women have aching backs.

- You're still constipated.
- You've got heartburn and indigestion indignities, such as bloating, burping, and flatulence.
- You don't seem to be racing to find bathrooms as often to urinate. (Don't become too comfortable with this turn of events. Your need to urinate will increase again in the last trimester as the baby grows bigger and the pressure on your bladder makes you want to go all the time.)
- You get dizzy and feel lightheaded.
- Your nose is stuffed up and drippy on occasion. It feels as if your allergies are working out of season.
- You are incredibly hungry and find yourself desperately seeking treats at all hours of the day and night.
- You crave sleep although you are not quite as sleepy as you were back in the very beginning of your pregnancy. If you are finding it difficult to sleep face down now because of your growing belly, you may be frustrated.
- You get headaches. Hormonal changes are probably the real culprit here, although anxiety, fatigue, and hunger can also make your head pound in ways you've never known before. If you get migraines, they may either become your worst nightmare now or disappear completely. Ask your practitioner for her or his recommendations for medicine to relieve them. Don't take aspirin.
- You notice changes in the color of your skin, specifically a dark line down the center of your belly (*linea nigra*) and splotches on your face (*chloasma*).
- You are still sweating after all these weeks because of your speedy metabolism. Even the palms of your hands get over-heated at times.
- Your breasts are still growing and nipples may be darker yet. In fact, your breasts produce colostrum, the first fluid your new baby will receive from you if you are breastfeeding. Made up of water, proteins, minerals, and antibodies to protect a newborn, colostrum is thick and yellow early in

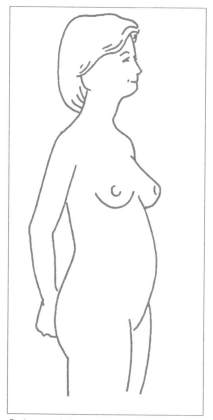

During month five, your breasts might increase—dramatically—and the womb becomes level with your navel.

pregnancy but becomes clearer and thinner later. You may have noticed some of it leaking from your breasts, especially when you are making love or are sexually excited.

- You've gained at least six pounds.
- When you lie down or sit for a rest, your stomach doesn't stop moving, as your unborn baby tries out new movements and develops muscle. Late evening is when fetuses are ordinarily most active.
- Your fingernails may be soft and brittle because of the increased level of hormones. Have your nails done by a professional manicurist.

For Your Information: Hair Hints

You put your hand to your hair and it doesn't feel the same anymore. The texture of your hair changes. If it used to be oily, now it's even more oily. You've got more of it, too.

Although hair is definitely dead, all those extra hormones and nutrients in your bloodstream can make it silkier and improve its condition. You'll want to change your hair care routine. Not only has the texture changed from normal, oily, or dry to some other category altogether, but also you may have noticed that it feels thicker. In fact, you probably do have more hair on your head than you did five months ago. When you aren't pregnant, all women tend to lose about 100 hairs a day. This is normal. When you are expecting, the hair stops falling out until after the birth. Your thickened mane is not the result of growing more hair but of not losing as much each day.

Take care of your hair. Play with hair care products. Experiment with new shampoos and conditioners, for instance. If you've always used a shampoo for normal, oily, or dry hair, it's time to try something else. Don't stick with the same brand for months and months. In fact, don't rub the conditioner into your scalp. Try applying it only to the ends of your hair before rinsing.

- Wash your hair more frequently but be careful not to dry it out.

- There's no reason why you can't have your hair dyed. Even though your hairdressers may be operating under the assumption that dye is worrisome for pregnant women, you don't need to worry, according to Dr. Howard Berk. Transdermal (through the skin) medications are absorbed very slowly. The amount of time the dye is on your head is short by comparison.

More Symptoms That Say: "Yes, You're Normal"

Your skin may be glowing from extra oils being released. Some women see blemishes disappear. Pregnancy, especially during this second trimester, can do wonders for your overall look. If you have sensitive skin, however, all the hormones combined with tension can contribute to breakouts, rashes, allergies, dryness, or extreme oiliness. Oh that shiny nose! Your skin is probably never either better or worse than now.

Are You Seeing Stretch Marks?

Almost all expectant mothers develop what are euphemistically called stretch marks. Breasts, hips, as well as the abdomen, are trouble spots. I did. My friends did, too. Yes, we freaked a little at first. What were these pink or even reddish indentations or streaks? Would they be there for life ever after?

Stretch marks are the response of your skin to the steroids that your body is putting out. You see this happen when someone is given cortisone and develops stria or white lines on the skin's surface. Young women who are just starting to menstruate can develop stretch marks, not from the skin doing any stretching, however, but from the steroids they are producing. Creams and oils will not make stretch marks disappear, but time will.

Dark Lines and Patchy Blotches?

You may notice changes in skin color, specifically that dark line down the center of your belly (*linea nigra*). You've always had a white line that runs from your belly button down to the top of your

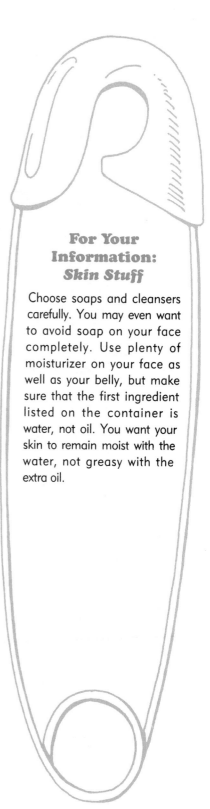

For Your Information: Skin Stuff

Choose soaps and cleansers carefully. You may even want to avoid soap on your face completely. Use plenty of moisturizer on your face as well as your belly, but make sure that the first ingredient listed on the container is water, not oil. You want your skin to remain moist with the water, not greasy with the extra oil.

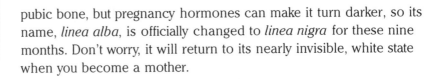

pubic bone, but pregnancy hormones can make it turn darker, so its name, *linea alba*, is officially changed to *linea nigra* for these nine months. Don't worry, it will return to its nearly invisible, white state when you become a mother.

A Mask of Pregnancy?

Because the change in skin pigmentation shows up across your cheeks, nose, upper lip, and forehead, *chloasma* is commonly called "the mask of pregnancy." For dark-skinned women, the "mask" may appear lighter and in light-skinned women, the pigmentation is darker. Researchers suspect that it is caused by an extra sensitivity to all the estrogen circulating in your body. Have you noticed that your freckles are darker? Are your moles standing out more, too? Estrogen is sending the pituitary gland in your brain a message to release more of the melanocyte-stimulating hormone (MSH). The MSH makes your skin secrete more of the skin pigment known as *melanin*.

What to do about chloasma?

- Be patient. It will go away. Yes, if you've got a case of chloasma, you are certainly not very happy about it, but the good news is that this overheated state of skin pigmentation will gradually disappear after the birth.
- Don't go out in the bright sunshine without a hat as well as lots of sunscreen. Buy a sunblock especially for your face with the highest number SPF you can find. Direct sunlight can make discoloration worse.
- Check your vitamins. Are you getting enough folic acid? There may be a relationship between the B vitamin, found naturally in fruits, green leafy vegetables, dried beans, peas, and whole-grain products and skin pigmentation problems. Folic acid, the synthetic form of folate, is undoubtedly in your pregnancy vitamin arsenal, but when you discuss chloasma with your doctor, you might want to mention this aspect. Recent reports indicate that all women of child-bearing years need at least 400 micrograms and during pregnancy, you ought to have at least 800 micrograms a day. Not

only is folic acid critical to your health but also a lack of this essential nutrient has been linked to brain and development problems in babies. In a new folic acid fortification program required by the Food and Drug Administration (FDA), manufacturers are being asked to add this vitamin to flours, breads, corn, grits, rice, and even noodle products. Some breakfast cereals are already fortified with folic acid.

In Your Doctor's Bag of Tools and Tests

Your routine urine tests may indicate a high level of sugar in your system, which could mean that you are developing a type of diabetes known as *gestational*. If you've been feeling fine and sailing through these weeks, this news may come as a shock. Don't freak out yet. Sugar in your urine, especially during the second trimester, is not unusual. Fifty percent of all expectant moms show up with excess sugar. Your fast-growing fetus is demanding lots of nutrients and your biochemistry simply isn't keeping up with the demands. Not enough insulin is being produced and the excess sugar is ending up in your kidneys. In many cases, a second urine test will show that this imbalance has disappeared because your body starts producing more insulin to take care of the excess sugar. If high sugar levels appear after a second urine test, your doctor may order a blood test to confirm the condition and a glucose tolerance test (GTT) to see if your problem is more serious. Glucose is simply a type of sugar, but too much of it in your body is not a good thing for you and your growing baby.

You may be asked to keep track of fetal movement. All unborn babies are different and their activity can be erratic. When you are really busy you may not even notice the kicking, shoving, twisting, and turning. In fact, fetal activity becomes more clearly defined and active only after Week 24 and up to Week 32. Some doctors suggest that you try to keep track of the movement by counting kicks or movement of any kind at certain times each day. Consider good strong kicks, as well as swishing, fluttering, rolling, and turning. Your doctor will undoubtedly have suggestions.

Is It Diabetes?

- Keep in mind that the way your body metabolizes sugar always undergoes a big change when you are expecting. In fact, normal pregnancies bring on a diabetic-like state, so a case of gestational diabetes now does not mean that you will have full-blown diabetes after the birth.
- Your doctor may arrange for you to speak with a certified diabetic educator so you can learn how to check your glucose level at home with a store-bought monitor.
- You may be placed on a special diet for diabetics.
- An ultrasound can check the growth and well-being of your baby. When it is uncontrolled, gestational diabetes alters the way your baby grows, increasing the size but hindering the maturity. In other words, you can have a big baby not physically ready or prepared for life. By measuring the fetal movement and breathing patterns, an ultrasound will ensure that growth is right on target for size.

Need More Folate? Eat These Foods!

Food	Serving Size	Amount (Mg)	% Daily Value
Chicken liver	3.5 oz	770	193
Breakfast cereal	½ to 1½ cup	100–400	25–100
Braised beef liver	3.5 oz	217	54
Lentils, cooked	½ cup	180	45
Chickpeas	½ cup	141	35
Asparagus	½ cup	132	33
Spinach, cooked	½ cup	131	33
Black beans	½ cup	128	32
Burritos with beans	2 burritos	118	30
Kidney beans	½ cup	115	29
Baked beans (pork)	1 cup	92	23
Lima beans	½ cup	78	20
Tomato juice	1 cup	48	12
Brussel sprouts	½ cup	47	12
Orange	1 med	47	12
Broccoli, cooked	½ cup	39	10
French fries	Large order	38	10
Wheat germ	2 tbsp	38	10
Fortified white bread	1 slice	38	10

(*Source*: Food Values of Portions Commonly Used, 16th ed., Kurtzweil, Paula, FDA Public Affairs, "How Folate Can Help Prevent Birth Defects," 1998, http://www.babybag.com)

The old approach was to relax, lie back, and try to look at the clock in the middle of a busy day to catch your unborn baby kicking. The object was to note at least ten movements, checking the time before and after, and writing it down. Experts believe that fetuses sleep in short bursts of twenty to forty minutes at a time, so if you were unlucky and caught yours during a neonatal nap, you were to try counting kicks later. Within a two-hour span, you were told to catch at least ten moves. However, Dr. Howard Berk has a more modern approach for busy women anxious to count kicks. "In the world today, what woman has time to lie down to check her kick counts? Only when she is ready to fall asleep is this possible. During the day, she's either working, she's got other kids to take care of, she's providing transportation for her family, or she may even be writing a book. An active woman can't spend time lying down watching the clock."

Instead, choose four hours in the morning when you are active. You should feel four separate groups of movements within that time frame. You don't have to count specific kicks. What you are looking for is fetal movement.

Dr. Berk cautions, "I also don't recommend this until the end of a pregnancy or if a complicated situation exists. If you don't feel any movement at all during that four-hour period, then call your practitioner. A sonogram can be employed to watch the movement as well as a non-stress test. In the meantime, to try counting kicks at only twenty weeks is really too soon. You've almost just begun to feel the baby and what those little pats mean. Start your own modern-day kick counting at the end of month seven."

You could be scheduled for a non-stress test (NST). This test, done to measure fetal heart rate, can be done at any time after your unborn baby's heart starts beating and is not necessarily scheduled for your second trimester. When you move, your heart rate speeds up and so does your baby's. These ups and downs in fetal heart rate are considered a good sign. You'll be on a bed or examining table attached to the same kind of fetal monitor used during delivery. The belt is strapped around your abdomen. For about twenty minutes, every time you feel your baby move, you'll push a button. In

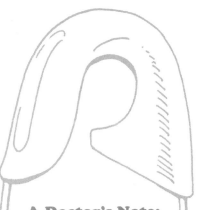

A Doctor's Note: The Yellow Cab Syndrome

"The non-stress test is similar to what I call the yellow cab syndrome. If you are crossing a busy street, and a yellow cab is approaching you, your pulse rises. In much the same way, the fetus's pulse rises when there is sudden movement. It will go up approximately 16 beats. If you want to wake up the baby or increase the pressure, nipple massage will be effective. Or, simply having the pregnant woman drink orange juice. Most babies begin to kick after they have had something to eat."

—Howard Berk, M.D.

some situations, the monitor detects the movement without your pushing a button. What the testers—and you, too—want to see is your baby's heart rate going up and then back down. If there is no change at all with the activity, fetal distress is suspected. Sometimes, a buzzer or vibrations are used to wake up a sleeping fetus. If so, your NST includes a fancy extra called *vibroacoustic stimulation*.

Your doctor may ask for a Biophysical Profile (BPP). When you have an ultrasound combined with a non-stress test (NST), you end up with a BPP. Fetal heart rate, muscle tone, body and breathing movement, as well as the amount of amniotic fluid are all noted and included on your chart. Did I say breathing? Well, of course, your baby isn't breathing real honest-to-goodness oxygen yet, but he or she is making all the right moves. The fetus gets oxygen from your placenta. A score of 8 to 10 is normal. The test will take about a half-hour.

Other tests to determine how your baby is growing may be scheduled. If everything is proceeding along normally, your doctor may not even mention some of the other tests that make it possible to see your baby's progress.

However, if there is any concern about the baby or if you are still pregnant at forty-one or forty-two weeks, the first thing you'll have is the non-stress test. If that test is not reactive, you could be asked to have a *stress test*, or *oxytocin challenge test* (OCT), in which mild contractions are induced to see how the baby responds. The hormone pitocin will be injected to start the stress test. If the baby cannot maintain his heartbeat during a contraction or if the heartbeat falls, this is an indication for immediate delivery, according to Dr. Berk.

Doppler velocimetry can measure blood flow to the umbilical cord. *Fetal electrocardiography* checks fetal heart rate. In a *fetal scalp stimulation*, someone actually puts pressure or pinches the unborn baby's head. Sometimes, a sampling of blood is taken.

Backache Essentials

- Sit down. Standing aggravates the ache. If you must stand on your feet longer than you would like, put one foot up on a box or pile of books.
- Pencil in time to lie down as often as you can. Make it a commitment you keep.
- What kind of shoes are you wearing? Low heels may offer relief even more than flats.
- Skip grocery shopping, or if you must, have someone else cart your bags. You want to avoid lifting heavy objects. When you must lift, bend from your knees, keeping your back as straight as you can. Bend your knees and stand with a foot on each side of the object you want to lift so you use both arms and divide the weight. Bring the object closer to your body. Don't reach up for heavy objects on high shelves.
- Find chairs with good back support. If you are working in an office or at a computer, a chair that makes your back feel great is an absolute must. Can't change your chair? Carry a small pillow with you to place at your lower back for support.
- Don't sleep flat on your back. Turn sideways and put a bed pillow between your knees. A mattress that is too soft can also make your back hurt.
- Schedule a professional massage. Make a regular appointment something on your "must-do" list from now to the end of your pregnancy.
- Stand tall and be aware of your posture. With the new weight right out front, it's only natural to overarch your back and push your abdomen out even further. Drop your shoulders and keep them back. Tuck in your backside. Lift your chest and rib cage.
- Go slowly when you get up after sleeping or lying down. Turn to your side, push up with one arm, and use your thigh muscles.

I Was Wondering . . .

I can't sleep soundly anymore. My favorite sleeping position is on my stomach and I just can't get comfortable anymore. What do you suggest?

Let's face it, your whole life is changing, not just your sleeping routines. Your inability to snuggle into an old, comfortable sleeping position in bed may be just the first of many upheavals in the next few months. After the baby is born, you will be moving into new bedtime rituals, too. Some tips for now: Treat yourself to new pillows and try several arrangements to make yourself more comfortable. Look for one of the new full body pillows. Open the window to allow more fresh air into your bedroom if the outside temperature is pleasant. Take a warm bath before you go into bed. Put a pile of magazines beside your bed so you can read even if you can't sleep. Don't choose any serious reading material, however. Have a light snack in the evening so hunger doesn't wake you.

Don't drink any liquids after your dinner except a glass of warm milk. This tactic may cut your trips to the bathroom, and the tryptophan, a sedating substance in milk, might help. Volunteers in a research study on the sedating effects of milk fell asleep faster, awakened less often during the night, and spent more time in deep, dreaming states. You need the calcium in the milk, too. So does your growing baby. Meanwhile, stop counting the hours you sleep and consider how you feel instead. Fatigue is part of all pregnancies, so napping during the day is just fine. Exercising can also help tire your muscles so you are ready to fall asleep. If you find yourself tossing, turning, and uncomfortable about even being in bed, get up and do something that is fun.

I seem to notice pregnant women everywhere now. Why am I so aware of them now?

Yes, this does happen and I remember thinking that there must be an epidemic of pregnancy in my neighborhood. There really was no local baby boom in my case and there may or may not be in your own. Your heightened awareness of all the other women expecting babies probably comes from your own highly sensitive state. Now that you know what it feels like, you automatically seek out other women experiencing the same ups and downs. When you couple this very special wavelength you are on with the fact that you are putting yourself in situations where you are more likely to meet and see more mothers-to-be—doctor's offices, pregnancy classes, hospital tours—it's no surprise that pregnancy seems to be popping up all over in your life.

My husband and I are thinking about taking a vacation now. Is the fifth month a good time to go?

Middle months of pregnancy can be an excellent time to escape from your routine, especially if you are no longer experiencing morning sickness and you have more energy. Later, in the last trimester, a vacation may not be as much fun or even advised.

Mention your travel plans to your practitioner especially if you plan to be far away from your home or out of the country. You may need to take a copy of your prenatal medical records with you and you will want to obtain a list of do's and don'ts. Get up and move around every couple of hours, especially if you expect to be in transit for a long time. If you are going by car, stop and walk around. On a plane or train, get up and go up and down the aisle. Think comfort when you pack and dress. Put crackers, snacks, water, or juice in your travel bag. Eat balanced, nutritious meals when you are away so you don't upset your already sensitive digestive tract. If you've been plagued with constipation, take foods with fiber along as well as plenty of water to help you stay as regular as possible. Put a box of prunes in your suitcase, for instance. Don't use this tremendous opportunity to eat out as a chance to pig out on poor foods.

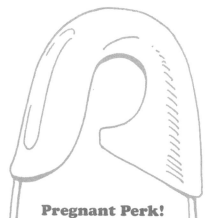

Pregnant Perk!

Take Advantage of Body Rhythms

Now that you have a bit more energy and you are less fatigued, look for your prime time. There may be twenty-four hours in every day, but your mood and energy level can never keep up around the clock. Some women are at their peak between 10 A.M. and 2 P.M. You know your body best even now. Devote those peak periods to important tasks. Save your mindless routines (or napping) for when you know you'll run out of steam.

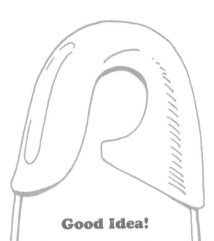

Good Idea!

When you sit down, elevate your feet high enough so the blood rushes back into your body. Can you raise the bottom of your bed mattress? Even a few inches can help. Don't sit cross-legged. Buy and wear support stockings or leotards. Ask your practitioner for recommendations.

I've never had varicose veins before. Why should I be developing them now?

During pregnancy, the pressure inside the veins in your legs is three times what it is normally. If you are overweight, if you are up on your feet for hours on end, if this is your second or third pregnancy, or if the tendency runs in your family, then those poor veins are likely to rebel with swelling and pain. You need to improve circulation, so blood doesn't collect in your legs, making them ache and your feet puff up. Start exercising by gently circling your ankles and feet whenever you can. In fact, take a good look at your regular exercise routine. Is there something else you can be doing to help your blood circulating? For instance, swimming is excellent. In the water, leaning against the side of the pool, raise your leg to hip level and make small circles in front and to the side. Then, move to the next leg. Other water aerobics are wonderful for varicose veins. Even if you consider yourself a nonswimmer, try it. You don't have to dive in and start swimming laps right away. The water will support your pregnant weight and make you feel more buoyant than when you are on land.

Is a vegetarian diet okay for my baby's growth?

Sure. Just be careful that you are eating a variety of protein-rich foods and lots of fruits and vegetables daily. Vegetarians who also avoid milk as well as eggs, ought to pay special attention to protein servings and calcium intake. If you are careful, your baby will be getting all the necessary nutrients. You may also need to take an iron supplement, however, because human beings have a difficult time absorbing the iron they need from plant sources. If your practitioner has recommended prenatal vitamins, iron is a mineral you are getting daily. I'd recommend a serious discussion with your practitioner or a nutritionist to talk about your diet and how it will affect the baby's growth.

News reports of food poisonings make me awfully nervous, especially now that I'm pregnant. Should I be worried?

Outbreaks of food contamination can be scary now that you are eating for two. Millions of bacterial food poisonings are reported every year and you certainly don't want to become one of these statistics or someone making news headlines because of a disaster. Here are a couple of factors to make you rest a little easier. Most cases of food poisoning are not fatal, even though they can make you feel positively terrible. Although the media may frighten you into thinking that eating out can be dangerous to your health, you are more likely to suffer from food poisoning as a result of careless handling and meal preparation at home. The foods most likely to become contaminated are meat, poultry, fish, shellfish, and unpasteurized milk.

Arm yourself with some defensive maneuvers to protect you and your unborn baby. When you prepare food, wash up always and often. Hands, kitchen counters, and utensils should always be immersed in hot, soapy water before, after, and even in between meal-making steps. Toss that damp, used, dish cloth right into your laundry bin because it can promote bacterial growth. Wash sponges thoroughly in hot water and don't keep them forever. Never let food sit on a counter or dinner table for more than two hours if the temperature of the food is between 45 and 140 degrees Fahrenheit. Be careful when you fill your plate from a buffet table or smorgasbord. Refrigerate or freeze leftovers promptly. If food is discolored or smells funny, dump it. If a can or container has been leaking or is swollen, throw it away.

Certificate of Birth

Finding the Top of Your Uterus

Your expanding belly will be measured and palpated (gently poked, pushed) again and again. By thirty-two weeks, the fundus, or the top of your uterus, is well above your belly button and putting pressure on your ribs and diaphragm. Do you realize that by the end of your ninth month, that versatile organ will have expanded in size to 500 times what it was before you got pregnant? In weight gain alone, your uterus goes from about an ounce and a half to thirty ounces.

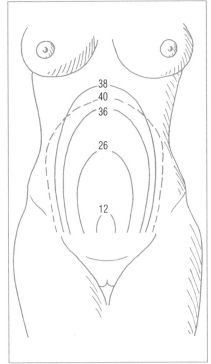

Throughout pregnancy, the height of the fundus will rise, and then fall just before delivery. Numbers shown indicate weeks of pregnancy.

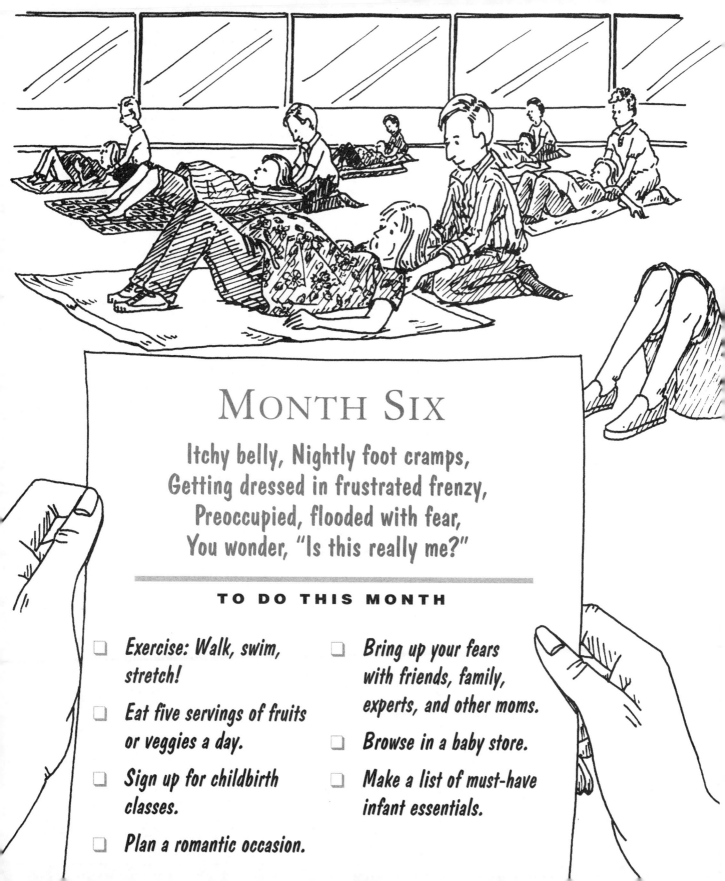

MONTH SIX

Itchy belly, Nightly foot cramps,
Getting dressed in frustrated frenzy,
Preoccupied, flooded with fear,
You wonder, "Is this really me?"

TO DO THIS MONTH

- ☐ *Exercise: Walk, swim, stretch!*
- ☐ *Eat five servings of fruits or veggies a day.*
- ☐ *Sign up for childbirth classes.*
- ☐ *Plan a romantic occasion.*
- ☐ *Bring up your fears with friends, family, experts, and other moms.*
- ☐ *Browse in a baby store.*
- ☐ *Make a list of must-have infant essentials.*

Your rapidly growing belly may be the most obvious statement to the world about your pregnancy. You are harboring a little human being and this monumental truth can overwhelm you emotionally on occasion. Flooded with thoughts of your baby, upcoming labor and delivery, and of becoming a mother, your moods may swing wildly. On down days, I could see no bright side at all to life. When the stretching, itching skin of my belly became the subject of conversation and my husband trying to cheer me up with a joke, I didn't want to get *it* (his humor) or get happy. Yes, of course, I'd soon be able to clean the lint out of my navel with ease, but why was that supposed to be funny? While people around me contemplated snowstorms, preparing their taxes, work-related deadlines or real world anxieties, I could hardly stay focused on tasks immediately in front of me. My ups and downs took me for wild rides.

When I was down, I'd even worry about whether or not I could be motherly enough. I had never been one of those women who peeked at other people's babies in carriages or offered to babysit. What would happen to me after my own baby arrived? Would these instincts really come naturally or might I fail in the nurturing department. The first time around, before my son was born, I questioned my future life as an individual. Would I still be able to be a separate person? Or, would I turn into my own mother?

What Are You Feeling Emotionally?
Unreasonably Teary?

I can remember crying about an overripe banana at breakfast.

Fearful?

A friend recalls receiving a piece of junk mail announcing that one out of every eighty-seven children was born with some dread deformity. She promptly walked to the nearest school and at recess, counted the kids who came out to play. When she reached number eighty-six, she paused and wondered, would her baby be number eighty-seven?

Fearless?

On my up days, when the entire world of pregnancy seemed conquerable, I felt powerful, untouchable, or, to use a better word in this context, impregnable. Run around the park? Sure! Paint the baby's room? No problem! Finish every last item on my "to-do" list and still find time to call an old friend at night? Of course. Plan a party for the week before my estimated delivery date? Why not!

Frustrated?

"How are you feeling?" can become the most worn-out phrase in your daily encounters with the outside world. Everyone, sometimes even strangers, ask you over and over again. Some walk right up and feel your belly. Most don't really want to know about your abdominal gas, signs of varicose veins, your aversion to apricots, or craving for pasta. Polite . . . you are supposed to be polite, even when these outsiders come up with the most intimate answers or snippets of advice that you are supposed to follow. Never having been a person who found it easy to discuss things like hemorrhoids, weight gain, or up-close and personal biological matters, I found this spotlight on my health emotionally uncomfortable. You may, too. Keep in mind that you have a perfect right to feel violated and emotionally vulnerable. You can also simply say, "No thanks" to the suggestions from strangers.

Fixated on Strange Symptoms?

Unusual side effects with only spotty explanations can establish a place in your mind and refuse to let go. My ears ached whenever I put on a pair of pierced earrings—even the expensive and hypo-allergenic kinds. After my doctor could find no rational, medical reason and after I had asked in all the right circles, looking for an applicable old wives' tale, I came across someone else who had suffered the same slight agony. Bonnie, a friend with three children, assured me that after each of her deliveries, her ears, and her ability to wear earrings without ear-ringing, returned to normal.

Soooo . . . Other Pregnant Women Have These Symptoms, Too:

- Tender breasts
- Fatigue
- Occasional dizziness
- Frequent urination
- Constipation
- Stomach as well as intestinal gas
- Bleeding gums
- Runny nose, stuffy sinuses
- Headaches
- Vaginal discharge
- Signs of varicose veins
- Feeling stuffed
- Weird changes in skin and hair
- Mildly swollen feet, ankles, face, or hands
- Flutters and burbling sensations from deep inside your womb

Shocked?

One morning during my sixth month, I found myself standing in the aisle of a crowded train. Liberated as I had become, I saw nothing unusual about not receiving an offer from a gentleman for a seat. It was winter and warm in the car and as I took off my coat, the train went through a dark tunnel and I glimpsed my reflection in the opposite window. Why, I looked like a pregnant lady! It was me. Me? Oh God! Could it really be me? Then, I quickly wondered, if it really was me in such a pronouncedly pregnant state, why *didn't* someone offer me a seat?

Scared?

It's only natural to be afraid. You are heading into unknown territory. You may be lucky and have the shortest labor and delivery on record. Then again, you may spend hours confined to a small space in a situation in which there is no turning back. All those authorities—experts, authors, currently and formerly pregnant women—try to sound comforting, as they put the pain of childbirth into some kind of self-controllable package you will manage. Yet, thousands of years of history, literature, and books tell you otherwise. Terrible screams, agonies of birth, pangs of labor, even anthropological references that describe pains "like fine electric needles outlining one's pelvis" during labor, can scare you (Margaret Mead said that). Victorian women used to put on the shroud of death at their first labor pain because they had a 50 percent chance of dying.

Am I trying to make you more frightened? No. What I want you to realize is that your fears are very legitimate, so don't let anyone tell you to set your worries aside. Instead, get prepared. Yes, you are going through a time of vulnerability, dependency, and personal upheaval, but the chances of childbirth killing you or your baby are really minimal. You are going to survive and thrive. The pain? Let's just say, it's do-able and you'll learn what to do when it starts. If I can do it, so can you! In the meantime, start collecting childbirth tales from all the women in your family. From this homework assignment, you may find similarities that will prepare you in a very personal way.

Oh Baby . . . Inside Secrets Now

- About thirteen inches long, your unborn baby is gaining pounds exponentially fast from this point forward. He or she may be up to two pounds by the end of this month.
- Organs are developed, although the little body is lean with not much sign of fat yet.
- The face is thin, so the eyes look big and prominent.
- Eyelids are starting to open. Eyebrows? Yes.
- Scheduled for an ultrasound this month? If so, be prepared for E.T. Seriously, just a glimpse of that little face on the screen may lead you to suspect that somewhere in your family tree is an alien from a distant planet. Don't worry, this lost-in-space look changes dramatically in the next few months.
- Sweat glands are forming just beneath the surface of the skin.
- Alternating bursts of activity with periods of rest, your baby experiments with all the amazing movements that can be made with arms and legs. Sit still and concentrate on what may be happening inside. When you sense the moving, kicking, turning, twisting, see if you can detect which part of the fetal body is doing all the pushing and shoving. Is it a foot? An elbow? A head? Or a backside?
- Fingernails are forming.
- He can cough. She can hiccup. Drinking too much of the warm amniotic fluid can bring on these very naturally human reactions. Meanwhile, amniotic fluid filled with precious nutrients is excreted from the fetus's body as urine.
- Because hearing is becoming even more fine-tuned, the sound of your voice or certain types of music are more soothing than ever before.
- Frowning, squinting, pursing lips, this little being even has fingerprints now as well as definite footprints.

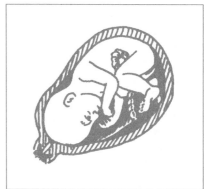

By week 24, the eyes seem to bulge because the face is thin. The skin of the torso becomes thicker as well.

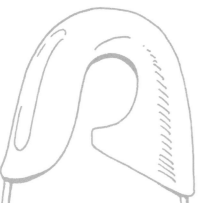

U.S. Army Cure for Leg Cramps

So you aren't in the army? Well, that's no reason to discard a rather ingenious cure for leg and foot cramps. It was the United States Army that came up with the warm water/cold floor connection, according to Dr. Berk. "When soldiers would march around in the hot fields, they would lose their calcium and end up with leg and foot cramps. It was in one of their manuals that I saw the remedy that works quite nicely for anyone, including a pregnant woman, with a muscle cramp."

Let's Get Physical
You're Normal If . . .

- You've gained at least ten pounds and your womb has moved well up above your navel.
- Your upper arms seem bigger. Shirts are snug and not just across your bust line. The cause? Probably water retention, not fat.
- Your breasts are still growing and you may need a bigger bra again. Treat yourself to something lacy or black. You deserve a break today.
- You are becoming convinced that you may be carrying more than one baby. (Relax. Unless multiple births run in your family, you were taking a fertility drug before you became pregnant, or your doctor and an ultrasound have confirmed the existence of multiple babies, you probably can count on one little child arriving in about three months.)
- You get cramps in your legs and feet especially at night. I would be in bed, finally comfortable in a nice cozy position when suddenly, a weird, pulling, painful cramping in the arch of my foot would force me up and out. These cramps plague some women in their legs and can be caused by an imbalance of calcium and phosphorus in your body. Simply increasing the amount of calcium in your diet may not be sufficient, however. According to Dr. Berk, you need aluminum gels or any aluminum-based antacid that will increase the absorption of calcium in a form that will prevent the cramps. Look for Amphi-gel or Rolaids. In the meantime, when a cramp strikes, stretch your leg or point your toes down. If your leg cramp is in the calf, stretch your toes up towards your head. Grab your toes and pull on them. That will stretch the calf muscles out. Of course, it's always great to have a massage. Stand up and walk to the bathroom sink. Wash your hands with warm water. Dr. Berk explains, "This is an electrical potential because the difference between the warm water on your hands and the cold

floor on your bare feet helps to relieve and straighten out the cramp."

- Your belly itches. As the skin on your stomach stretches and pulls tighter and tighter, the itchiness may increase. Use a mild skin cream regularly to keep your skin soft and pliable.
- You're still breathless and insistent about opening windows everywhere you go.
- Your shoes don't fit anymore. You may not believe this, but with each of my children, I gained a full shoe size. Not every expectant mom is forced to buy all new shoes, however. Your shoes may feel snug because you are retaining water in your feet. The joints in your feet actually do spread during pregnancy because the hormone relaxin is loosening everything up in anticipation of delivery. That includes feet, unfortunately. Buy new shoes for now and think comfort first. Forget heels. Choose sneakers or walking shoes. Look for styles that will let your toes and joints spread out with ease. Sit down and put your feet up as often as you can.
- You experience twinges of pain in your lower abdomen from time to time. Unless you are feeling downright sick, with a fever, congestion, chills, or severe pain, your abdominal sensations are probably just related to stretching ligaments and joints. Your uterus is growing rapidly now and causing everything else to be pulled along with it.
- Your lower back still aches. Those muscles and ligaments are so stretched and loosened now that your risk of back injury is high. Your center of gravity is continuing to shift forward, too, which puts a strain on your lower back.
- You've lost your old stamina. The demand on your cardiovascular system is greater in this second trimester. You may lose steam or energy as a result. Old exercise routines, for instance, aren't quite as easily completed. The urge to quit halfway through is most compelling.
- Your face may be puffy. That's water, too. Speak with your doctor if you are concerned. Regular check-ups should be ruling out any serious concerns connected with fluid retention.

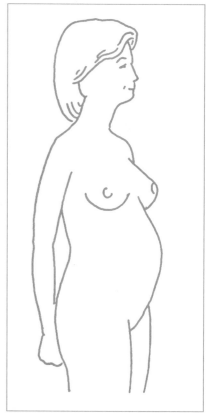

You might be gaining about one pound a week during this month, as your belly is rapidly enlarging.

You Should Worry If . . .

Your Doctor Says That You Are Showing Signs of Preeclampsia

Also known as *toxemia*, *preeclampsia* is a complicated, pregnancy-related version of high blood pressure or hypertension, which is more common in first-time mothers-to-be after Week 24. Other signs include: a quick jump in weight gain (from water retention, not baby growth); swollen ankles, feet, or hands; traces of protein in your urine sample; a blood pressure reading of 140/90; a persistent headache; blurry vision; and abdominal pain. Preeclampsia is serious, but treatable. You may end up in bed, either in the hospital or at home. You'll be drinking fluids, watching your sodium or salt intake, and may be put on medication to bring down your high blood pressure. Only a small percentage of pregnant women develop preeclampsia, but it is important for your doctor to keep these symptoms in check before they take you headlong into what is known as *eclampsia*. If your blood pressure increases to 160/110 or higher, you risk damaging your nervous system, having a seizure, going into a coma, destroying your kidneys and your circulation. Developing a full-blown case, though, is extremely rare for a woman under a doctor's care. However, if your symptoms of preeclampsia remain in your third trimester, labor may be induced or a cesarean section could be recommended. Most women with mild preeclampsia do just fine and blood pressure returns to normal after birth, sometimes within the first day of their baby's life.

You Are Diagnosed with an Incompetent Cervix

Normally in pregnancy, your cervix remains tightly closed until the onset of those first labor pains. If someone is discussing an incompetent cervix with you, it means that there is concern about the growing baby and womb putting enough pressure on your weak cervix to open it and cause a miscarriage. Most miscarriages occur in the first trimester, but an incompetent cervix can be cause for concern throughout pregnancy and especially in the second trimester when the baby is not ready to survive. If your cervix has been quietly thinning without any apparent contractions, then the doctor may notice this during an examination. Vaginal bleeding can also be a sign of danger.

An incompetent cervix can be traced back to a number of reasons: a genetic weakness, previous births, prior surgeries, especially abortions, as well as exposure to DES (diethylstilbestrol) when you were in your own mother's womb. If you are carrying more than one baby, you are more likely to have an incompetent cervix, too. Surgery to stitch the cervix tightly closed will be done almost immediately with a diagnosis of incompetency. "It is an emergency," explains Dr. Howard Berk. "If one of my patients walks in and tells me she has a little watery discharge, I'll examine her and if she has an incompetent cervix, she'll be sutured immediately. Then, in any subsequent pregnancy, once this diagnosis of incompetent cervix has been made, the suturing can be done electively about the twelfth to thirteenth week." These sutures will be snipped before your delivery date.

One of the signs of an incompetent cervix is a blood-tinged discharge, so it's important to call your practitioner if this happens in your middle trimester. A test called a *hysterosalpingogram* can indicate an incompetent cervix and will also show adhesions in the womb and tube blockages. The official name for the suturing surgery is the *Shirodkar procedure*. Other treatments and steps are also available and you can be certain that frequent exams will be on your calendar. Sometimes, bed rest is prescribed, as well as abstinence from any sexual intercourse. An appliance called a *pessary*, which is inserted into your vagina, may also be recommended to support the uterus. In the meantime, be certain to take note of any strange pressure, discharges, or symptoms in your lower abdomen or vagina.

You Experience a Heavy, "Won't-Go-Away" Pain, Not a Muscle Cramp, in the Calf of Your Leg

Unlike ordinary, troublesome cramping, this kind of pain refuses to disappear within a few minutes. You may see swelling, redness, and the area could be tender to your touch. Perhaps the nearby veins look more prominent than usual. Known as *venous thrombosis*, this condition is a blood clot that occurs once or twice in every one hundred pregnancies. You are more likely to develop

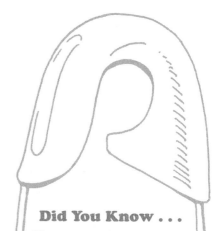

Did You Know . . .

Those annoying cramps at night in your calves or legs could be caused by lack of vitamins? Are you getting enough calcium?

Your need for iron doubles when you are expecting?

The joints and ligaments in your feet will stretch and can send you into the next shoe size?

Having sex can be full of surprises in pregnancy?

clots when you are pregnant. Not only is your body getting ready to stop any excess flow of blood during birth by strengthening its clotting ability but also because of your enlarged uterus, blood flow can be impaired and circulation slowed. One of the symptoms of venous thrombosis is a pain in the area where you flex or stretch your leg. If the area is tender, swollen, or you have any other unusual symptoms, don't wait to seek some medical expertise.

You Have Any Vaginal Bleeding of Any Kind

Bleeding at any time during pregnancy should be reported to your doctor, but now that you are in your second trimester, the blood could be a sign of an impending miscarriage, an incompetent cervix, or a problem with the placenta. Occasionally, the placenta has implanted itself close to, or partially covering, the cervix (*placenta previa*). As your pregnancy proceeds, this could become the kind of problem that sends you to the hospital and calls for a cesarean section at delivery time. An ultrasound can indicate placenta previa. However, even low-lying placentas do move upward as growth continues, so you may simply be sent to bed if your bleeding is light or intermittent. Extra iron, lots of vitamin C, close medical supervision in a hospital setting, and possibly blood transfusions, can keep your baby safe until you reach at least thirty-six weeks in the pregnancy when delivery is safer.

Vaginal bleeding and/or abdominal cramping can also indicate that the placenta has begun to separate from the wall of the uterus, a more serious condition called *placental abruption*. Definitely an emergency, placental abruption survival odds have become better because of good medical care, hospitalization, and early diagnosis. Bed rest has changed the odds of survival dramatically in recent years. Almost all mothers and babies can win this battle beautifully.

Pregnant Body Basics
Shape Sorting

Some of us carry our unborn babies high, some low, some all over, some hardly at all. (We've all heard those tales of moms wearing their own clothes right into the hospital and then accepting

Academy Awards two weeks later while wearing strapless, slinky gowns. Hmmm.) After watching and recording hundreds of pregnancies in northern New Jersey, I'm convinced that there is little way to predict the physical spin your pregnancy will put on you. This wide variation in pregnancy shaping may not have even dawned on you until now. Where are you going with your body now? Did you ever believe you would have so little control? Honestly, most books depend on a single female silhouette to show the shape of things to come. We all know that this is just not true. In fact, no one knows it more intimately than you do now.

Out of the Mouths of Mothers . . . and Fathers

- "Your own pregnancy shape is always a surprise when you spot yourself in a mirror or store window. For some reason, I guess because it comes on slowly month by month, you can't easily adjust to that big belly when you look at it squarely. Inside, you are still slim or in the same body you had before."
- "Perhaps the strangest thing about the public nature of pregnancy is that many women seem to take it all in stride. I kept waiting for my wife to bite some belly-rubber's hand off, but she never did. For some men, however, this touching business can bring out feelings of anger. 'Nobody touches my woman!'"

New (Or Soon-to-be) Body Basics . . .

Ahem . . . Can You Find Yourself Among These Fruits and/or Balls?

Just for fun, see if you can put yourself into one of these categories:

Are You Carrying a Low-Slung Basketball?

Your unborn baby won't have to drop at that very last stage of events just before delivery and exit. If this is you, your uterus is

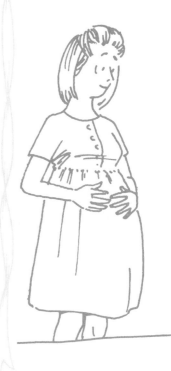

still low. In fact, it may not reach up to be tight against your rib cage ever. You could be all out front, causing some strangers to suggest that you are definitely carrying a girl while others insist you are most definitely having a boy. You may be so low that your waistline is nearly visible and you are tempted to wear a belt some days.

Is It a High Ball, However?

The good news: regular, nonmaternity underpants may fit fine right until almost the last moment when your baby heads down into the pelvic area. Unfortunately, your rib cage is gently but insistently being pushed up. Get ready for your breasts to rest on your belly, causing a strange but not necessarily disagreeable sensation. Unfortunately, you can't wait to take a deep breath.

How About a Watermelon?

If you wanted to recreate the look of this pregnancy after the delivery, you could probably buy a watermelon some summer day and strap it to your waist. Not possible? Of course not. Seriously, your pregnant bulge begins right under your breasts and extends down in a gentle oval to your pubic bone.

Do You Look Like a Pumpkin?

Pumpkin-shaped pregnancies can be emotionally painful because you can appear to be expecting something all over, not just in front. Your growing pumpkin may extend down to the tops of your thighs. A rear-view glance can make you cringe. Don't torture yourself. You will be able to get out of this patch sooner than you think.

What About a Ripened Pear?

Bottom heavy, you may be worrying about your thighs a lot these days because that's where this pregnancy is hitting you hard. No one ever told you that weight gain in pregnancy was not necessarily confined to the abdominal area.

Are You Turning Into a Refrigerator?

Even watching your calories and nutritional needs closely doesn't seem to help reign in this metamorphosis of your body. If you are gaining your weight all over—upper arms, bust, belly, and legs—blame it on a genetic connection. Did your mother put on pregnancy weight in the same way? Relax. Don't accept the grief from the nurses and doctors who refuse to believe you are sticking to a sound diet plan. Yet, don't use the refrigerator shape as an excuse to go wild. After all, you will want to slip back into your old shape in a few months.

I Was Wondering . . .

Are sugar substitutes okay? Can they cause problems during pregnancy?

Unless you have diabetes and need to control your sugar intake, you really don't have a good reason to consume a lot of artificial sweeteners. However, if you have grown accustomed to the taste of sugar substitutes, you don't have to worry about side effects or problems. There are three sweeteners commonly used today: aspartame, saccharin, and acesulfame K. *Aspartame* has been clinically tested and is safe to use during pregnancy for everyone except women who have a condition known as *phenylketonuria* (PKU). Both the Food and Drug Administration (FDA) and the American Academy of Pediatrics agree that aspartame is quite safe for both you and your baby. *Saccharin* passes straight through your digestive system without change and even if some does cross the placenta and reaches your developing baby, experts say there is no harm done. In fact, the American Diabetes Association recommends that expectant moms with diabetes use saccharin. In research studies of the sweetener known as *acesulfame K*, no toxic effects came up.

Why do I need to take iron supplements? My doctor has recommended lots of iron, but I think it's upsetting my digestive system.

Your need for iron doubles when you are expecting a baby because of your own expanded blood supply as well as the placenta's requirements. Your unborn baby is also storing iron that will

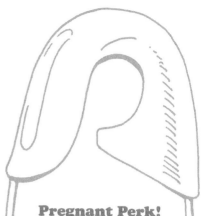

Pregnant Perk!

Stop Running to Answer Every Urgent Request.

A ringing telephone, a doorbell, or the sudden demand of an impatient co-worker can make you jump— no matter what else you may have been doing. Even in mid-bite, midsentence, or mid-nap, you may feel obliged to answer all such demands for your time. Urgent requests aren't always important. The next time you start to rush, think: Is this really important or could it wait?

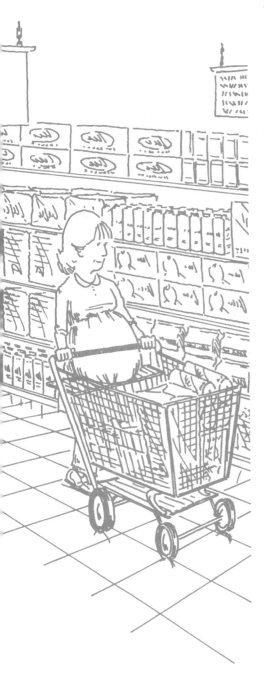

last for the first few months of life outside your womb. You've just got to get at least 30 milligrams a day. The baby won't suffer if you are not getting enough iron, but *you* will. You will end up with *anemia*, a deficiency in your red blood cells, a condition that can make you feel tired. Your baby is drawing iron from you. An insufficient supply of hemoglobin makes it harder for your blood to carry oxygen to the baby, puts a strain on your heart and can lead to physiological stress.

You are absolutely right about the effect of iron on your digestion. Take your iron-enriched prenatal vitamin supplements between meals with plenty of water or along with a fruit juice rich in vitamin C to eliminate some side effects of constipation, diarrhea, and nausea. The ascorbic acid in orange juice, for instance, enhances the absorption of iron. If constipation is a problem, add prune juice to your diet. Stay away from milk, tea, or coffee when you take your iron supplements. Some of your iron supply can come straight from foods. Add liver and red meat to your shopping cart regularly. Meats, fish, or poultry are high in iron, as are enriched and whole-grain breads and cereals, green leafy vegetables, legumes, eggs, and dried fruits. In the meantime, if the extra water and fruit juices don't help your indigestion, try taking your pills at bedtime to reduce stomach and intestinal flare-ups. Perhaps you can sleep through it.

I can't get enough ice cream, but I just heard about another mother who's been craving things like clay, coffee grounds, cornstarch, and candle wax. Could this be true?

Yes. Your craving for ice cream sounds normal. Sometimes, the hunger for certain foods is one of the first signs of pregnancy. Some women go for salty snack foods or pickles, which may indicate the increased need of the body for minerals. Cheese and ice cream are hot items, too. Who hasn't heard the stories of obliging husbands being sent out in the dark of night to buy half-gallons of mint chocolate chip ice cream?

When I was pregnant the second time, I could eat citrus fruits, especially grapefruits, all day. When I was thirsty, I drank gallons of pink grapefruit juice. The craving for bizarre substances such as clay, laundry starch, cornstarch, paint, ashes, ice chips, coffee grounds, paraffin, or baking soda is different. The woman you mentioned is suffering from a phenomenon called *pica*. Although cases of pica have turned up in the medical literature since the sixth century, no one knows exactly why it happens in pregnancy. Some experts have toyed with a connection to a woman's iron deficiency. Strangely enough, pica shows up more often in expectant mothers who live in the Southern United States. At least one old folk tale states that eating clay will help labor and delivery, take away headaches, get rid of swelling, and make a baby beautiful. If you don't give in to the cravings of pica, it is said that your baby will arrive with a disfiguring birthmark. Not only is this a silly myth, but it is also dangerous. Eating such awful stuff can result in an intestinal obstruction, preeclampsia (pregnancy-induced high blood pressure), a premature birth, and blood disorders. A baby born to a mother who indulged in plaster or paint ashes can also have lead poisoning. Contaminated clay can introduce intestinal parasites into the mother's body, too. If you know this woman, please make sure that she gets medical attention for her cravings right away.

My car's seat belt is so uncomfortable. Can it hurt my unborn baby?

Although you may not feel like buckling up across your pregnant belly, you really must. Automobile accidents are a leading cause of death among expectant moms, and the American Academy of Obstetricians and Gynecologists (ACOG) recommends wearing a belt whenever you are in a moving vehicle. Seat belts are designed to accommodate 400-pound men, so you should be able to adjust the straps to suit you and your baby well into your ninth month and still be comfortable. Don't worry about the belt putting pressure on your uterus. The baby is protected in the sac of amniotic fluid as well as the thick wall of the uterus that actually has several layers of muscle, tissue, and fat. However, to adjust the belt and still be comfortable, put the lap portion under your uterus and fix the shoulder strap so it lands between your breasts. Try to keep the belt snug with no more than three inches of slack. If you end up in a crash, you and your baby will end up in the car and not thrown onto the road. Did you know that most accidents take place within twenty-five miles of home?

I was so sick and so exhausted during my first three months that having intercourse became unthinkable. Now that I'm a bit back to normal, I can't help but think that we are hurting the baby. Could this be true?

No matter what kind of love life you had before you became pregnant or how many children you already have, sex is almost always full of surprises when you are expecting. As my friend Kay Willis, a mother of ten, always says, "The climax is just the beginning." Take ten close friends who are moms and you'll soon find ten very different tales. For some lucky women, the boost in hormone levels, the heightened sensitivity, and the feeling of voluptuousness actually increase sexual drive. These couples have more fun than ever. For others, each trimester brings a new set of romantic obstacles.

During those first three months, especially if you have morning sickness, sex can be quite unappetizing. Nausea can kill desire pretty quickly. If you are so sleepy that you have been fantasizing happily about slipping into a coma, making love slips down your list of preferred activities, too. Emotionally unstable, wondering what the heck is going on with that old, familiar body, lots of women find it hard to let go and become sexually excited. Breasts are tender. Vaginas are congested with extra blood flow. You've got white, sticky discharge to deal with and gaseous upset as well. Other inhibiting turn-offs to any romantic interludes: burping, bloating, sweating, breathlessness, sneezing, stuffy head, sudden leg and cramps, swollen feet, and constipation. If the hero in your life can get both of you past these obstacles, he may find himself awkwardly uncomfortable trying to maneuver around your growing abdomen and into a space that may seem to be the habitat of the baby now and not belonging to either of you at all: the womb at the end of your vagina. If the fetus is active, things can get even more complicated psychologically for some expectant parents.

Be patient with each other. You are not going to harm your unborn baby by making love, especially during this second trimester, unless you are already in a high-risk category. Although the uterus can contract during an orgasm, it won't bring on labor, and if your pregnancy is normal, sex is quite safe. The uterus is sealed at the cervix with a thick mucus plug. Reports of infection or miscarriage as a result of sex are scattered and more speculative than scientific. Only in that last month before your due date should you proceed with caution. Yet, don't worry. As Dr. Howard Berk says, "Some couples have been waiting all of their lives to have sex without using a condom. During pregnancy, most often infection does not occur and if it does, it is usually normal vaginal flora and therefore a condom would not work as a preventative." Other reasons to restrict your lovemaking include: vaginal bleeding, a history of miscarriage or premature labor, or a diagnosis of placental problems. If you are carrying more than one baby and heading closely into the home stretch (last eight to twelve weeks) intercourse may become something to save until after labor and delivery.

Try new positions. Be creative in your quest to remain intimately involved with each other. You may find, as many women do, that once they are over the hill of the early months, desire for sex increases. Plan ahead and go on real dates with each other so you can sit down together and talk about your lives without real or imagined interruptions. Wear something that makes you feel feminine. A change of scene may be essential, in fact. A chat at your kitchen table is not romantic when you are looking at a pile of dirty dishes to be washed and put away. Above all, keep talking.

In the last six to eight weeks of pregnancy, your practitioner may have additional recommendations about making love. If you feel comfortable discussing the issue, be sure to bring it up at your next appointment. Some professionals are reticent to raise the issue of sex unless you initiate the discussion.

Should I quit my job in a dental office now? I've begun to worry about exposure to chemicals, X-rays, and hazardous substances.

You do need to be careful because a dentist's office can be unsafe for your baby now that you are pregnant. Are you a dental technician who must deal with X-rays on a regular basis? If so, then definitely bring up your concerns with your employer as well as your practitioner. Exposure to radiation is dangerous, and so are chemicals like the nitrous oxide in laughing gas and the mercury, or even mercury fumes, used in some dental offices.

Even if you are just sitting in front of a video display terminal at a computer all day, you could be putting yourself in an unhealthy situation because of low-level radiation. Ask for a list of possible pollutants in the office. You don't need to go crazy, but you do need to proceed with caution. Sit down with your practitioner and ask for his help in sorting through your options.

Even though my medical insurance is paying for most of our bills now, I've been wondering about how expensive it will be to raise a child. How much does it cost?

In a report prepared by Philip J. Longman for *U.S. News & World Report*, estimates went as high as $1.45 million for a middle-income family raising a child to age twenty-two. Longman's figures were based on United States Department of Agriculture data which are updated annually. To the federal numbers, however, were added the cost of a college education and the lost wages many mothers experience when they drop out of the job market even for a short while. Higher income families spend as much as $2.78 million and if you are in the lower financial bracket, you can get by with $761,871 in costs. Longman explains that he didn't even consider the ticket for extras like "soccer camp, cello lessons, and SAT prep." Just buying clothes for your child until he or she is eighteen years old may strain your budget. Boys need $22,063 worth of duds and girls will be 18 percent more (or another $3,871.34).

Curious about the costs of pregnancy and childbirth? Longman says that a normal, no-risk pregnancy with twelve prenatal visits to the doctor's office and vaginal delivery averages about $2,800 in the U.S. Health insurance turns out to be a financial cost-saver because uninsured expectant moms actually pay more for normal pregnancies and deliveries: $6,400. If you end up with a cesarean section, the bill will be about $11,000 and complicated, high-risk pregnancies go up to $400,000. Every day a premature baby spends in the hospital adds up with a range of $1,000 to $2,500 per diem.

A friend who is also expecting just mentioned a condition called "uteroplacental insufficiency" or UPI. What is it?

When the placenta is unable to nourish the fetus, some experts refer to the condition as *uteroplacental insufficiency*, or UPI. The placenta, which is desperately important for your unborn baby's survival, must supply enough blood and nutrients to the baby and be able to carry away waste materials and carbon dioxide. If you are suffering from some kind of physical disorder (high blood pressure, diabetes, preeclampsia, chronic kidney disease), your placenta may not be up to the task. Some theorists believe that UPI is the real reason for many late miscarriages as well as babies born with brain damage or obvious fetal growth retardation.

What's a doula? My next-door neighbor hired one to help with her labor and delivery last year.

A *doula* is a woman who has specialized in helping couples make childbirth a pleasant and productive affair. The word itself is Greek and means "a woman caregiver of another woman." Not exactly midwives, doulas do receive formal training in easing and shortening labor. Not a new idea at all, doulas exist in many cultures all over the world and used to be more popular even here in the United States. Some studies do show that working with a doula

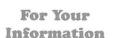

For Your Information

The word *placenta* was coined back in 1559 and comes from a Latin phrase meaning "circular cake." According to David M. Lima, M.D., in Yale University's Department of Obstetrics and Gynecology, the tissue separating your fetus from your placenta is so thick that nutrients and oxygen can be exchanged but not blood. In your third trimester, the placenta looks like a disk-shaped organ, measures about twenty centimeters in diameter and is two to three inches in thickness. Its maternal side is attached to your uterus and the fetal side has the umbilical cord connection linking you to your unborn baby.

can change labor significantly, making it shorter by several hours, reducing the likelihood of the need for anesthesia or of a C-section delivery. If you think you'd like to hire a doula, contact the Doulas of North America, 1100 Twenty-Third Avenue East, Seattle, WA. If your husband is frightened about coaching you through the birth, even after he completes childbirth classes, a doula might be a nice option. Marshall Klaus, M.D., famous for his theories about mother–infant bonding immediately after birth, explains that a doula, "will never take over or attempt to control the birth. We make the mistake of thinking that a father can take a birthing class and be prepared to be the main source of support and knowledge for the entire labor. That's just unreasonable. A doula can reach out to the man, decreasing his anxiety, giving him support and encouragement, and allowing him to interact with his partner in a more caring and nurturing fashion."

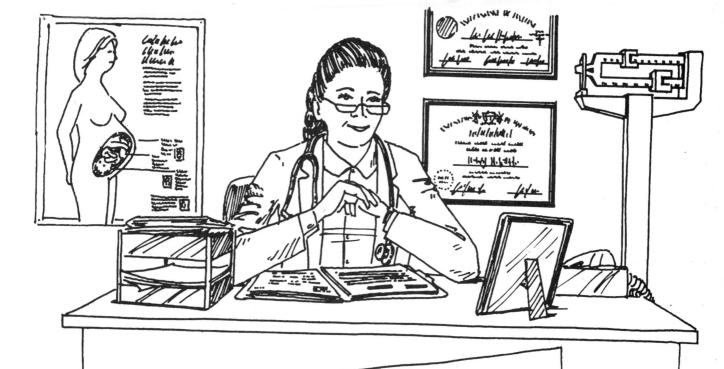

MONTH SEVEN

Planning ahead, You discover more childbirth lingo:
natural, prepared, Lamaze, LeBoyer, LaLeche . . . ,
And personally meet up with Braxton-Hicks

TO DO THIS MONTH

☐ *If you haven't already signed up for childbirth classes, do so now.*

☐ *Go over important issues with your doctor.*

☐ *Schedule a tour of the hospital or birthing center where you plan to deliver.*

☐ *Learn all the signs of premature labor.*

☐ *Post emergency phone numbers—your doctor's, for instance—prominently near the kitchen and bedroom phones.*

L ike a hungry diner surveying the scene of a smorgasbord, you are now facing some pretty incredible choices as you start into this seventh month. Hungry for good advice and counsel? Of course. If all goes well and you reach your ninth month safely, soundly, and still pregnant, the choices you make regarding classes, labor, delivery, and birth will affect you, your baby, and the way you begin your lives together. Don't duck these issues, allowing other people to make your decisions. Will it be Lamaze, LeBoyer, natural, prepared, medicated, or wide awake? Will you be in a hospital, birthing center, or stay home? Other questions about labor, delivery, and life in general loom larger than ever now. In discussing this last trimester, Elizabeth Whelan, M.D., caught the conflicting emotions clearly, "You are future oriented, suddenly interested in catalogs of nursery furniture and baby clothes, but with a nagging uneasiness about buying things for someone who has not yet entered the world." Books and medical advice can make you crazy. Remembering her own experience, Whelan admits, "After going through five or ten of the basic volumes for expectant parents, we began to feel that we knew more about the fallopian tubes, progesterone, and cervical dilation than we really cared to."

What Are You Feeling Emotionally?

Confused? Twenty years ago, when I was midway through a series of Lamaze childbirth preparation classes and seven months' pregnant, a discussion about hospital policies concerning brand-new mothers and their newborns sent me into a confusing spin for a few days. The instructor, a nurse at the hospital where I was planning to give birth, informed the six eager, pregnant couples that new babies would be taken from the parents in the delivery room and deposited at the hospital nursery where they would remain under the watchful eyes of nurses and the hot lights of a technology far superior to a mother's warm breast. No ifs, ands, or buts about it—that was hospital policy. No babies allowed in the recovery room. What's more, she explained, you might not meet the new member of your family for another four, six, or even twelve hours, depending on the time of day or night you had delivered.

On the phone with my obstetrician the next day, I started to cry. "You are obviously having a bad day," she said to me in a rather officious voice. "Moreover, you are reading far too much for your own good."

When I finally dried my tears, I decided to find a new doctor and another hospital. It had struck me that other people don't always know best. Three days later, after gathering reports and recommendations on obstetricians and hospitals from sympathetic friends and co-workers, I met my new OB. "Brinley," he said matter-of-factly at our first meeting in his comfortably cluttered office, "it's your baby and wanting that time together immediately after the delivery is not unreasonable at all."

In the years since my own private battle with a hospital policy, many institutions have come to agree that whenever medically possible, the feelings of mothers, babies, and fathers should come first—and hospital policies second. What's important for you to realize is that you do have choices. Before you go to your regular check-up this month, be sure to make a list of your concerns and questions. Don't assume that you understand exactly what your doctor is planning. Ask.

Oh Baby . . . Inside Secrets Now

- Your unborn baby has reached a landmark in development by this seventh month. Chances of survival outside your body get better and better now, day by day.
- Your baby is getting close to four pounds in weight and sixteen inches in length. These gains in size will be phenomenal during this last trimester.
- The top of your uterus is halfway between your belly button and your breastbone and it's cramping all your internal organs, especially your stomach, intestines, and diaphragm.
- Beneath red, wrinkled skin, fat is accumulating, which makes your baby appear flesh-colored. The lanugo, a downy

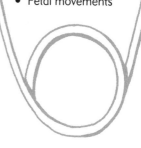

Soooo . . . Other Pregnant Women Have These Symptoms, Too:

- Tender, growing-even-bigger breasts that may leak sticky colostrum
- Lack of stamina
- Achy, swollen feet and puffy ankles, face, and hands
- Backaches
- Breathlessness, lightheadedness
- Frequent urination
- Insomnia
- Constipation, indigestion, heartburn, and stomach as well as intestinal gas
- Hemorrhoids
- Runny nose, stuffy sinuses
- Headaches
- Vaginal discharges
- Stretch marks and varicose veins
- Skin flareups and hair hassles
- Braxton-Hicks contractions
- Fetal movements

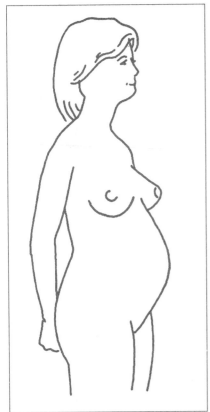

Your womb is moving up your torso and is now halfway between your navel and your breastbone.

covering of hair, is shedding and real hair on the head will soon start growing.

- Dramatic developments in the thinking part of the brain take place this month. A seven-month-old fetus feels pain, can cry, and behaves almost like a full-term infant.
- When stimulated by light or sound, your fetus will respond. Eyes are open with real eyebrows and eyelashes, too.
- Your ability to feel all the activities inside depend on your build, the position of your placenta, and the baby's size. Have your mate place his hands gently up against your abdomen during the early evening hours or when you suspect the baby is likely to be up and about. Sometimes the baby will react to the sense of touch from your outside world.
- Your unborn baby has a strong sense of taste and some experts suspect that fetal taste buds are actually stronger in the womb than after birth.
- Missing a critical ingredient known as *surfactant*, the lungs wouldn't be quite operable in the real world yet. Surfactant keeps them from collapsing in between breaths. Yet, surfactant can be increased in the fetus by giving intramuscular steroids to the mother prior to her delivery. Also, when membranes rupture or other forms of stress occur, surfactant increases. Chemical surfactants can be used after birth to help with respiratory distress.
- That slight repetitive jarring you sense could be hiccups, which have been known to continue for up to a half-hour.

Beginning Lessons in Childbirth Lingo

The language spoken by people in the childbirth community is dotted with a curious mixture of medicalese, French, and European imports with a sociological/psychological flavor. If you haven't been pregnant before or close to someone who has been, some of the terms may be puzzling. If you have a question, ask for an answer, no matter how silly you think it sounds or how professionally offi-cious the expert—nurse, doctor, midwife, resident, intern, neonatolo-gist—in front of you appears to be. Some questions have already been answered and issues settled by this seventh month. Yet, a refresher on the basics is always nice to have on hand.

Birthing Options

Hospital Birth

Let's face it, hospitals can offer you all the equipment and the experts you may need. Drugs for pain medication, electronic fetal monitoring machines to track the progress of your labor and the baby inside, everything for emergency intervention will be right at your bedside or at least nearby. A couple of days' rest afterward in a clean, comfortable bed where you will be fed and comforted by nurses is also an option most women go for. While many hos-pitals try to hurry you out as quickly as possible after a normal delivery, you may be able to stretch your stay up to forty-eight hours. Ask for information about what your insurance plan pro-vides. First-time mothers also welcome the inside information and hands-on care and nurturing that are often available from obstet-rical and pediatric nurses.

Take the Tour

Even if this is the very same hospital where you've visited all your recuperating relatives for years and you know the gift shop wares by heart, don't skip the tour of the obstetric and maternity areas. You will quickly find out about family-centered activities, including visiting hours or policies for husbands and siblings. Word-of-mouth tips are worth seeking, so ask other moms who have deliv-ered at your hospital of choice.

Birthing Rooms

If you deliver in a typical hospital setting, you will labor in one room and just before the baby is ready to be born, you'll be trans-ferred down the hall to the delivery room or operating room. All this movement can come at a most inopportune time. There can be no worse feeling for a mom who has been in labor for many hours and who is ready to push out her baby than to be told, "Hold on a minute. We need to transfer you to the delivery room." I can remember being in a hospital corridor traffic jam of rolling beds when there really was no way to put a stop to the imminent arrival of my son.

In recent years, more hospitals have realized that moving a woman so close to delivery is not a very nice thing to do. Birthing rooms within the hospital setting are designed for low-risk pregnancies and if you and your doctor expect things to go normally, then ask for a reservation. You'll stay in one spot from beginning to end and these rooms usually offer homey touches. Find out if the room has a birthing bed or one with a split frame so that a bottom portion of the bed can detach at the time of delivery. It may be more comfortable for you, and the doctor or midwife can simply pull up a chair to help ease your baby out into the light of day. If you think you'd prefer this option, speak up early so your name will be added to the list.

Birthing Centers

Small, out-of-the-hospital facilities, these centers may be an option if you are in a normal, low-risk category. Occasionally, hospitals actually operate them on their own grounds or nearby. Sometimes staffed by midwives and obstetricians on call for emergencies, birthing centers can also provide your regular prenatal check-ups, childbirth classes, and some routine testing. If you are interested in learning more about birthing centers near you, contact the American College of Nurse Midwives, 1522 K Street, NW, Suite 1000, Washington, DC 20005.

Home Births

Some healthy, expectant mothers prefer to stay right at home during childbirth. If this is a path on your wish list, do make sure to plan ahead carefully. You need an expert—an obstetrician, experienced family doctor, a competent nurse midwife—to remain with you during your labor and delivery. You can't do this alone or with the single-handed assistance of your partner. Arranging a home birth is possible, but you may have to dig for resources and information. If you know of a mother who has successfully remained relaxed amidst her own family and familiar comfort zone for the birth of her baby, then ask about her arrangements and who handled the birth.

Foreign Phrases

Lamaze

Named after a French doctor, Fernand Lamaze, Lamaze classes are among the most popular classes in the United States today and can be taken privately or in a hospital. Set breathing exercises are stressed for each stage of labor, as are important relaxation techniques. Also emphasized to take your mind off your labor pains is the need to focus on something, almost hypnotically: a poster, your husband's face, a speck on the wall. As a Lamaze graduate, I can testify that it works, but not miraculously.

Dick-Read

Based on a British doctor's theories, these classes emphasize slow abdominal breathing and teach you how to focus on the feelings and signals your own body sends during labor. No need for outside props here. Supposedly harder to learn, this philosophy makes more sense to me now that I've been through the birth process twice.

Bradley

Denver obstetrician Robert Bradley developed this approach about fifty years ago, and childbirth people call it the "no-method" method. It's closer to Dick-Read than to Lamaze in theory. Classes teach couples how to relax and breathe deeply, but emphasis is on doing what comes naturally—the presence of papas to be, proper nutrition during pregnancy, and, most important, knowing all the options beforehand.

Home Births Are Not For Everyone

A home birth is not a good idea if you have any kind of long-standing health condition, including diabetes, heart or kidney disorder, a history of problems in childbirth, previous C-section, or if you go into labor prematurely. If you smoke or are carrying more than one baby, consider a hospital your safest bet, too.

LaLeche

Known by a Spanish phrase meaning "the milk," this organization was founded in the 1950s to promote breastfeeding in the United States when the practice was at an all-time low. Its local groups and books, which provide information as well as emotional support, are invaluable.

LeBoyer

To soften what he called the harsh trauma of being born, this French doctor advocated low lights in the delivery room, a warm bath for the new baby, calm voices, and soothing room temperatures. Some American physicians thought he was crazy back in the 1970s.

Class Ingredients: What Makes a Good One Good for You

If you've been feeling swamped by life lately, you may wonder why you need to take a class at all. Seriously, when your life is already busy and you are anticipating a time in your future when the concept of personal space disappears almost entirely, do you need to go out at night, commune with strangers, and listen to an expert describing a biological process that may be frightening you? Yes, of course.

The Ins, Outs, Ups & Downs of Childbirth Classes

Even if your library of reading material about pregnancy, labor, and the birth process is already overflowing, there is nothing more worthwhile than taking a class to prepare you and your mate for what lies ahead. Honestly, reading about pregnancy just isn't enough.

Here is what to expect.

- You will sit in a class, side-by-side with other pregnant couples near your own stage of development and drink in the emotional and physical support that can come from sharing experiences.
- You will listen to a trained childbirth educator. In my experience, these women (and yes, childbirth educators are usually female) who have decided to spend their lives helping

other people ease their babies into this world are often kind, supportive, and informative. You may find yourself asking questions you wouldn't dare bring up with your doctor.

- You will discuss all kinds of nitty-gritty details and fears with other couples forging ahead into the same great unknown as yourself. Even scary or weird dreams aren't off limits when you are among the instant friends you find in childbirth classes.

- You'll get detailed descriptions of the birth process. Sure, you skipped ahead to sections on labor and delivery and think you may know more than enough, but you don't. Aspects of childbirth that seem pretty clear on paper will become even more understandable and predictable when you are in a good class that suits you and your general approach to the kind of birth you'd like to have.

- You can pick up even more details about your hospital or birthing center.

- You must learn the best coping strategies, including how to breathe, relaxation techniques, all about anesthesia or other pain-controlling methods, and what each stage of labor will demand of your body and your mind.

- Your partner will learn how to offer you comfort. Classes, in fact, are especially important for fathers-to-be because they take the unknown out of the fear. My husband didn't panic or fall apart at the sight of blood because he had been told what to expect.

- You will learn to take one step at a time during labor and delivery because you will understand that those waves of contractions ebb and flow and certainly have a finish line with a happy ending.

Find the Right Teacher!

Although not all childbirth preparation classes are created equal, most will offer you a wonderful opportunity to learn, and by learning as much as you can, you'll

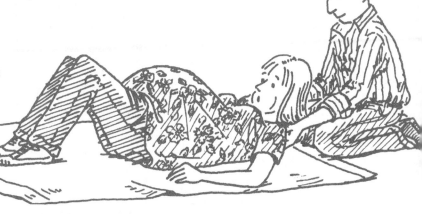

be less fearful and may end up having less pain. Some courses are intense, begin early in pregnancy, and try to take you through the whole nine months. Most hospital-based programs feature eight weekly sessions that start somewhere in the last trimester and are taught by a hospital employee who may spend quite a bit of time emphasizing in-house practices and procedures. Other classes are designed to be simple, one-night refresher courses for couples who simply want to brush up on ideas and techniques they learned for previous births. The growth of childbirth preparation classes since my mother's lonely birthing night has been absolutely tremendous. You may even want to sign up for baby CPR or safety classes, which will take you through all the emergency and first aid steps for your baby after birth. These classes aren't designed to scare you, but to prepare you. Don't miss this chance to start life as a mother fully prepared for the best, the worst, and all the in-between.

Do some thought work and homework first. Think about how you feel about being in pain and whether you will want to be given medication. If you are certain you will want to have an epidural, a type of anesthesia administered directly into the spaces between the vertebrae of your spine, you don't want to find yourself listening to an instructor who believes in an all-natural, no-drugs approach to birth. Your hospital may be the most natural route to a good class and possibly the cheapest. Call to find out when, where, and what kind of philosophy, if any, the educator espouses. Childbirth or Midwifery Centers offer classes. Ask your doctor or his staff for rec-ommendations. If you want to find a private class that may also be less crowded than the hospital route, you can call the International Childbirth Education Association (ICEA) at 612-854-8660 for the names of certified instructors in your area. According to information offered on their Web site (http://www.icea.org), ICEA "is a profes-sional organization that supports educators, parents, and other healthcare providers who believe in knowledge and freedom of choice in family-centered maternity and newborn care." Classes taught by an ICEA-trained educator, "typically focus on using as little medical intervention as possible but will provide you with an overview of all your options." For more information about ICEA, write P.O. Box 20048, Minneapolis, MN 55420.

Natural

An award for the most asked question must go to: "Will you be having natural childbirth?" By all rights, "natural" should mean nothing—no classes, no drugs, no hospital, no preparation. However, in most of today's birth literature, this term has come to mean an awake, aware, undrugged mother. It does not mean, as some people believe, a painless birth. (In childbirth, some women have a lot of pain and some have almost none.) Many women wrongly feel they've failed if they can't stand the pain and need a sedative.

Prepared

The best general word encompassing all the childbirth classes today is *prepared childbirth*, which can include lectures, exercise instructions, tours of maternity/obstetrics departments, and may combine several theories of how to manage labor.

Will it be Lamaze?

If it's a Lamaze class, named after the French doctor Fernand Lamaze, you will learn how to manage your pain using relaxation exercises and deep-breathing techniques. Dr. Lamaze, whose book *Painless Childbirth* was published in 1956, believes that all laboring women must have "a thorough preparation given by qualified people and a guarantee of peace, silence, comfort and the help of a qualified assistant during the whole of the labor." First witnessed by the doctor during a summer trip to Russia in 1951, the basis of Lamaze's work springs from a researcher named Ivan Pavlov, who believed that repetition and training could change thought processes.

With thirty years of experience as an obstetrician back in France, Lamaze was amazed to see women in Russia giving birth with virtually no pain because they had learned a practiced response, or a reflexive action, to use during labor and delivery. By concentrating intensely on a particular stimulus or action, you are supposed to be able to diminish your physical feelings. Let's call it mind over matter, and yes, it does work for some women, some of the time. I can attest to this.

Lamaze took the Russian ideas and taught his French patients a series of respiratory responses: slow breathing during the first stage

Don't Worry About Your Report Card

You don't pass or fail childbirth classes, so relax. There are no As, Bs, or Fs at the end of this term of instruction. Your goal is to learn as much as you can about childbirth and how to relax during the entire experience. If this is your first birth, you really don't know how your labor and delivery will feel, but let's face it, the odds and research indicate that you are going to have at least some discomfort. The expectant moms who are prepared are able to deal with it better. Even if you have some preconceived notion that you won't need anesthesia, you can always change your mind with no guilt. Seriously, rehearsing your approach to each stage of labor helps. Taking childbirth classes can shorten the length of your labor.

of labor, rapid breathing during the second stage, and a panting type of breathing as the child's head presents itself. His rather famous approach is called *psychoprophylaxis*.

If you sign up for an Americanized, updated version of Lamaze's course, the ICEA says you'll probably have twelve hours of instruction, be asked to bring your pillow for getting comfortable during practice sessions, and learn all about staying as pain-free as possible during the birth. However, Lamaze won't frighten you away from using anesthesia if this is a choice you find you must make. You'll get background information on epidurals and other anesthesias. More than two million parents choose a Lamaze childbirth class. For more information about the American Society of Psychoprophylaxis in Obstetrics (the official name for the Lamaze method), call 1-800-368-4404. You can also find them on the computer at their Web site, http://lamaze-childbirth.com.

How About Bradley-Based Coaching?

Another well-known approach to childbirth education is the Bradley method, which was actually the first to introduce the idea of husbands acting as coaches. Bradley's ideas are built on education, breathing, relaxation, and a husband-coach. If you find yourself speaking with a Bradley teacher, you should know that these educators always go through a regular recertification process, which is good news for you because they will be up-to-date on the latest in medicine and obstetrical circles. They will also emphasize the importance of a healthy diet and regular exercise. However, Bradley instructors try to ease you through the process with as little medication as possible, so if you've decided you want to leave your options open about anesthesia, you may want to reconsider a Bradley-based class.

Or, You Might Be Interested in Grantly Dick-Read

Another childbirth preparation crusader whose name you may encounter in your search of theories is Dr. Grantly Dick-Read, a British obstetrician who was determined to change the way women experienced so much pain during the birth process. His first book, *Natural Childbirth*, was published in England in 1933. Dr. Dick-Read believed that knowledge was power and got himself in so much trouble sharing his wisdom about labor, delivery, and other obstetrical intricacies that he was actually shunned by the British Medical Society, as well as the Anglican Church. He suspected that fear overstimulated the central nervous system and compounded whatever normal, natural pains a woman might be having during labor. Get rid of the fear and you may just be able to get rid of the pain. When he died, an obituary in the *British Journal of Obstetrics and Gynecology* called him "a crusader with almost too much fire in his belly," explains Dr. Elizabeth Whelan in *The Pregnancy Experience.* If you can get your hands on old books, you might also find it interesting to browse through Dick-Read's other works: *Childbirth without Fear*, *Natural Childbirth Primer*, and *Introduction to Motherhood.*

The Bing Option?

People in childbirth circles consider Elisabeth Bing, who has based her ideas on Dr. Lamaze's thinking, to be a leader in her approach to the use of psychoprophylaxis. Her book, *Six Practical Lessons for an Easier Childbirth*, is a classic, and she's known for her no-guilt, no-nonsense style. "You will learn to change your breathing deliberately during labor, adjusting it to the changing characteristics of the uterine contractions. This will demand an enormous concentrated effort on your part. Not a concentration on pain, but a concentration on your own activity in synchronizing your respiration to the signals that you receive from the uterus," she explains. "This strenuous activity will create a new center of concentration in the brain, thereby causing painful sensations during labor to become peripheral, to reduce their intensity."

Good Questions to Ask a Childbirth Instructor Before You Sign Up

Take these suggested questions, recommended by *The Baby Center*, "The Web's best for pregnancy and baby," to heart when you look for a childbirth educator. Designed for educational purposes, this Internet site is jam-packed with helpful hints. You can reach it at: http://babycenter.com.

Sign Up for Childbirth Classes Now

If you haven't started attending any classes yet, now is a great time to focus on the type you want to attend. Ask your doctor for recommendations. The hospital or birthing center where your baby will be delivered may have a special program that will also include valuable information about hospital policies. Outside consultants and classes also offer programs. Ask other expectant moms in your doctor's office for recommendations. Hospital-based classes may be more crowded and less personal. Private teachers can limit the number of couples and talk freely and frankly about hospital policies.

Also think about contacting your local chapter of La Leche League International if you are interested in breast-feeding.

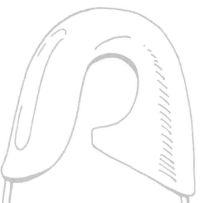

Pregnant Perk!

Learn How to Say NO.

Turning down someone who asks for a chunk of your time is never simple, but these suggestions may help:

• Say it fast before they can anticipate a yes. Hedging with "I don't know" or "Let me think about it" only complicates your life now, adding stress because you may want to beg off later.
• Be polite and pleasant.
• Offer a counterproposal.

1. Where did you get your teacher training? AHCC (Bradley)? ASPA (Lamaze)? ICEA? Other?
2. Why do you prefer this particular method? What are its strengths?
3. How long have you been teaching?
4. Have you yourself given birth using this method?
5. Where do you hold classes? How often does your class meet?
6. What can I expect to gain by taking your class?
7. How big are your classes?
8. Can I call you with questions between classes?
9. Do I have to do homework or prep work for classes?
10. How much does a class cost, and which insurance policies reimburse your services?
11. Can you recommend couples I can call for references?

Name _____ Phone _____
Name _____ Phone _____

12. What percentage of your students have unmedicated births? _____%
13. What percentage of your students have cesareans? _____%

About the Classes

1. Do your classes cover:

   Exercises and conditioning?
   Nutritional information?
   Relaxation techniques?
   Preparation for the labor coach?
   Breastfeeding instruction?
   Newborn care?

2. What are your thoughts on taking drugs for pain relief during labor?
3. Do you show childbirth videos?
4. Do you have written material for review?

Let's Get Physical
You're Normal If . . .

- Your stomach may be rumbling, bubbling, and reacting with violence to foods. Heartburn and gassy, bloated constipation are to be expected. Eat small meals if your appetite is large but your stomach is resisting. Skip the greasy fries and spicy foods. You'll feel better without indigestion. Eat as many fruits and vegetables as you can stand to ease constipation. Don't rely on laxatives, especially the ones that contain a compound called phenolphthalein. Along with your fruits and veggies, go with bran cereals, prune juice, and lots of water every day. Don't lie down right after eating because the uterus pressing on a full stomach can make you incredibly uncomfortable.

- Getting out of bed is getting difficult. While you have been trying out new sleeping positions in your efforts to get comfortable at night, a new sensation could be your inability to get up easily. Roll to your side and then push up with your hands. Don't try to sit up suddenly and put your feet quickly on the floor.

- You have swollen ankles and fingers. Called *edema*, this condition happens to almost everyone, during this last trimester. Your body is holding on to extra water. Have you noticed swelling in your ankles, especially during hot weather or at the end of the day? Show your practitioner, but don't worry. If your rings don't fit your fingers easily now, that's to be expected, too. However, keep in mind that dramatic swelling could be a sign of preeclampsia.

- Your skin may be sending you surprises. Stretch marks aside, your skin can also become extra sensitive and prone to a pimplelike condition featuring little red bumps on your stomach, thighs, and/or backside. Your face can also break out in a bevy of blemishes and prominent pimples. Hormonal changes are partially to blame, but so is the tension building up now. Breakouts, rashes, allergic reactions, extreme oiliness, and patches of flaky dryness are part of the pregnancy picture. Don't be alarmed. Bring up your dermatological concerns at your next office visit. Ask about creams, lotions, cleansing routines, and make-up.

- Your lower back could be complaining loudly and sending its painful message down your leg. Half of all pregnant women have back pain, especially as they move into this last trimester. If the pain in your lower back or buttocks is also sending its message down the back of your leg, you may have *sciatica*, or a swelling of one of the discs in your spine. The sciatic nerve could actually be pinched. The joints in your lower back are not functioning happily together because your growing uterus is forcing you into awkward positions. If you don't remember lifting, bending suddenly while trying to turn your body, or doing anything that might have brought on your pain, your dramatically changing posture could be the cause. Sometimes sciatica disappears when the baby changes positions. Ask your doctor about analgesics or safe drugs to reduce the inflammation. Put a heating pad on your pain. Inquire about special exercises.

- You aren't comfortable resting when you lie on your back. If you try to rest on your back during the last trimester, your enlarged uterus falls back and may decrease some blood flow to your heart. As a result, your blood pressure drops. You can't get comfortable. Lie on your left side and your circulatory system can work better.

- Your pulse seems to be faster than ever. Your heart is working overtime pumping blood not only through your body but also to the placenta and your unborn baby. If you take your resting pulse rate, it might be up ten to fifteen beats per minute. This is normal. Some women even develop a slight heart murmur when they are expecting as a result, but it will disappear after delivery.

- A stuffy nose is still irritating nasal membranes, making you sound funny and feel miserable. Ask your doctor for advice. Try to unclog your nose with a humidifier. The additional moisture may help the drying that can lead to nosebleeds.

Doctor's Note:
Sleepless Dads!

Some theorists believe that pregnant women should never fall asleep lying on their backs after the seventh or eighth month because of the risks from the uterus putting excess pressure on the veins carrying blood to the heart. In fact, this isn't something to worry about at all. "My mother never worried about it and she delivered a pretty good product," says Dr. Howard Berk. When you become uncomfortable on your back, even while you are sleeping, you will simply turn over to your side or change positions. There's no need for an expectant dad to stay up all night anticipating that his wife will need to be repositioned in bed. "When I have a patient who is markedly edematous or retaining an excess amount of fluid, or who has hypertension, I suggest that she lie on her left side from twelve to one during the day. The purpose of this timing is to decrease the production of a hormone called aldosterone, which regulates your electrolytes. This hormone is excreted when you lie on your back or when you sit as well as stand but never when you lie on your side. Aldosterone is also not excreted at night. Have you ever noticed that you weigh less in the morning than when you went to bed the night before? The reason is that you have turned off your production of aldosterone and you breathed your water out. If you have excess fluid in your body, lying on your left side at noontime will make you, as well as your husband, rest easier at night.

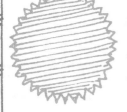

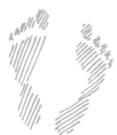

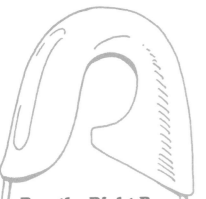

Buy the Right Bra

If you have never seriously had to think about bra sizes before, you may be realizing that buying the right size is no guessing game. First, measure your chest under your arm and above your bust. This measurement is the bra size, such as 32 or 34. Come up with an odd number? Go up one point, from 35 to 36, for instance. Next, measure your bust at the fullest point. This number will determine your cup size. If your bust number is 1 ½ inches larger than your chest figure, you are an A cup; 1 ½ to 2 ½ inches larger = B cup; 2 ½ to 3 ½ inches larger = C cup; 3 ½ to 4 ½ inches larger = D cup. For example, if your chest measures 34 inches and your bust measures 36 inches, your bra size would be 34 B.

- Your breasts are leaking and still growing bigger. Not only are your breasts heavier, but also they are more glandular and getting ready to feed your baby. In this last trimester, they may begin to leak colostrum, which is the nutrient-rich fluid that precedes real breast milk. Estrogen and progesterone are reaching record-high levels in your system and orchestrating all kinds of pregnancy-related changes. Your breasts may also need a lot of support, so look for a bra that has extra wide straps. If you are wearing a D cup or larger, this strap width makes good sense. Find a style that will cover your entire breast with full underarm and inner-cup support system. Some designs actually have soft-stretch elastic let-out darts in the front that can grow with you during these last months of pregnancy.

  If your breasts are really big, bend over when you fasten your bra to allow your breasts to fall into the cups' natural positions. You'll get a better fit. Also, make sure that the bra is snug around your chest. If it is too loose, it will ride up your back and push your breasts forward and down. If you are planning to breastfeed, consider buying your nursing bras now. Some can be adjusted for size easily.

- Worried about your varicose veins, you may be considering support stockings. Not a bad idea if you've noticed the development of varicose veins or if they run in your family. The extra support for your legs may be worth your investment, but be careful to buy the right size. These stockings have a greater tendency to slip down across your expanding waistline as you wear them. An orthopedic nurse I interviewed when she was nine months pregnant even opted for a doctor-prescribed type of surgical stocking that extended from her toes to her thighs and offered incredible support for her long working days spent on her feet. "I worked a ten-hour shift until my seventh month, and I really needed the support, so these surgical stockings were terrific. I would wear them underneath my regular stockings. We called them 'anti-embolism' (anti-blood clot) stockings in the hospital where I worked." Ask your doctor or midwife about them if you suspect you need extra support. "They really weren't hot, constricting, or too tight," this nurse added. Any surgical supply store carries such stockings, but you may need a prescription for a proper fit.

- You may experience Braxton-Hicks contractions, or false labor pains. Out of nowhere, you'll feel the tightening grip of the muscles surrounding your baby. Then, quickly, there is a gradual release. These are Braxton-Hicks contractions and can start happening after Week 20, continuing right up until your due date when the real act of birth begins. A big difference between a Braxton-Hicks and a real labor pain is that the cervix remains closed tightly.

  I used to consider these belly-tightening and cramping sensations a warm-up for the real labor yet to come; and in fact, they do seem to be nature's way of getting those muscles of your uterus ready for labor and delivery. For a few seconds, you may actually see your uterus harden, a strange sensation that can last as long as two minutes. Nearly painless and unlike real labor contractions, which have a predictable pattern and timing, the Braxton-Hicks variety are irregular and can hit you anywhere, anytime.

  Whenever I went swimming in the months before my daughter was born, I could expect a couple of embarrassing Braxton-Hicks, embarrassing because in a wet bathing suit, the hardening and contracting was actually visible to others around me. Was my unborn daughter unhappy about her dip into the cold water? Who knows? Yet, she was pretty predictable in her protest. If you are uncomfortable during a Braxton-Hicks, try changing positions. Sit down. Lie down. Stand up. In a swimming pool? Climb out and sit in the sun for a minute.

To check your unexpected contractions, lie down and put your fingertips on each side of your uterus. You may be able to feel the contractions better in this position. Keep still for a half hour. Sometimes, the uterus contracts so painlessly that you can't feel it when you are up and running around. Some experts recommend that all expectant moms who are in a high-risk category check for

Real or False Labor?

Real labor has a rhythm with contractions that occur very regularly and grow stronger and more frequent. If you are really going into labor early, you will be able to time the length of each contraction, as well as the calm interval in between this tightening or hardening of your uterus. You'll find a pattern. It could be one every ten minutes, one every twenty minutes, or one every hour. Pick up a pad and pencil and keep track if you suspect that a Braxton-Hicks could be the start of something more serious. Write down the exact time, how long the contraction lasts, as well as when the next one occurs. Time yourself for at least an hour. More than five within sixty minutes should send you to the telephone to alert your practitioner.

Are You at Risk for Premature or Preterm Labor?

If you've already had a baby prematurely . . .

If you are carrying more than one baby now . . .

If your cervix has been deemed incompetent . . .

If you have had a series of infections in your urinary tract or cervical area . . .

If your uterus is abnormal in any way . . .

If you've had an abortion before . . .

If you are under eighteen or over forty . . .

If you are obese . . .

If you are too thin and trying to stay that way for some misguided reason . . .

If you develop a fever with a really high temperature . . .

If you had surgery on your uterus . . .

If you have high blood pressure . . .

If you develop a kidney, liver, or heart problem . . .

If you are severely anemic . . .

If you are exercising much too strenuously . . .

If you are a heavy smoker . . .

If you are drinking alcohol or using drugs . . .

If you suffer a severe emotional breakdown . . .

If your mother took DES* . . .

Then, you may be at risk for premature labor.

* (DES stands for diethylstilbestrol and was once prescribed to women with obstetrical problems, diabetes, or vaginal bleeding during pregnancy. DES turned out to cause major problems for the daughters of women who were prescribed DES because it caused abnormal changes in their cervixes and/or vaginas. If you were exposed to DES in utero, then your practitioner will automatically place you in the high-risk category.)

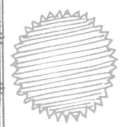

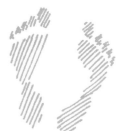

contractions in this way regularly. If you've experienced any bleeding since your fifth month, put this practice into your daily routine. You just don't want your baby's early arrival to catch you off guard.

Starting at the twentieth week, the uterus has a basic rhythm. The smooth muscle of the uterus is similar to your intestinal tract or the heart. All have peristalsis, or wavelike contractions. So painless contractions are not labor. Painful contractions are labor. The actual definition of labor, even when it is premature, is the onset of painful, uterine contractions that lead to a change in the cervix and end with the delivery of the baby.

Premature Labor
How Early Is Too Early?

Having a baby between the twentieth and thirty-seventh week of pregnancy is considered premature. Preemies can suffer from a wide range of neurological and physical difficulties and may simply be too undeveloped to survive at all. Stories of miracle babies surviving after spending only twenty weeks inside their mothers' warm, nurturing womb can make you cry with delight. However, even with all the advances in neonatology, you really want to avoid delivering before your term is up. In this, as well as so many aspects of life, timing is everything. Most pregnancies depend on a delicate hormonal, biochemical phenomenon that will allow labor to begin safely after the thirty-seventh week. Every effort to keep your baby safely inside will be made when premature contractions threaten to end your pregnancy too soon.

If You Are at Risk: Fourteen Mother-Friendly Pointers

1. Make your pregnancy as stress-free as possible. *Pssst. Don't tackle anything new. Don't plan elaborate parties, vacations, or encounters with difficult people. Pamper yourself. You are not being selfish. You are taking good care of your baby.*

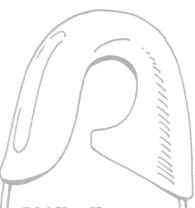

Did You Know . . .

The top of your uterus is halfway between your belly button and breastbone by now?

Half of all pregnant women have back pain?

By lying on your left side, your circulation will work better and sleeping soundly will be easier?

If your baby arrives prematurely, you both may be sent to the nearest "Level III" hospital with a neonatal intensive care unit?

2. Keep your doctor and medical team informed about any change of side effects or strange sensations.

3. Put emergency phone numbers and names in prominent places. Post them next to your kitchen phone. Carry them with you in your pocketbook.

4. Don't worry about appearing to be dubbed a nervous nilly by your doctor or nurses. You want to make sure that your body remains the warm, welcoming, nurturing environment it's been for the last six months because your baby needs to stay there as long as possible.

5. Build an at-home library of resource materials, including books, pamphlets, Web sites, and other moms' notes. Store your paperwork in one place so you can retrieve it when you need to research some particular side effect or funny feeling.

6. Don't keep your worries to yourself. Share your fears with your mate.

7. Skip strenuous exercise. You will get your body back soon enough.

8. Don't worry about getting all your chores done every day.

9. Think about taking an early leave of absence from your job if you are still employed away from home. Get a note from your doctor if you are worried about reactions at work.

10. Don't try to decorate the baby's room by yourself.

11. Stop lifting grocery bags and heavy objects.

12. Don't expect to shop non-stop unless you are browsing through catalogs.

13. Put your feet up and sit still every day as often and for as long as you can.

14. Be sure to discuss your sex life during regular office visits because the doctor may want you to abstain from inter-course until after the baby is born. Some physicians actually issue a no-sex warning after the fifth month for expectant moms in high-risk categories for premature labor.

Go to Bed

At the first inkling of any signs of impending labor, some practitioners will tell you to lie down and rest slightly on your side and

Good Idea:
Ask Your Doctor About the
Closest Level III Hospital

A Level III Neonatal Care Hospital will feature:

- Capability of managing even the most complicated, high-risk birth
- Transport, even by air, of the mother and baby to its facility or another hospital in its network. (You could end up in a helicopter, and these medical centers have heliports.)
- Every kind of testing imaginable.
- Fetal monitoring equipment
- Sophisticated surgical procedures even for the tiniest baby

- Amniocentesis
- Diagnostic ultrasound
- Genetic studies and counseling
- Special laboratory and pathology testing
- Neonatal intensive care units
- Educational programs for you as the new mom
- Special programs for expectant moms who are known to be at high risk because of a pre-existing health disorder such as diabetes, heart disease, or epilepsy
- A team of very skilled professionals at your service

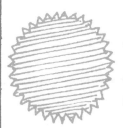

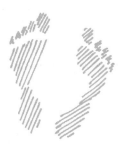

put a pillow along your back for support. Don't turn completely sideways because you may not be able to feel the contractions as definitively. Keep timing the contractions, noting actual time on the clock of the beginning as well as the end.

Premature labor will call for quick action on your part as well as your doctor's. Some doctors believe in a regimen of complete bed rest as well as drugs to relax your uterus from contracting. You could also end up in the hospital. Even if you remain home, you will be closely monitored. Drugs designed to stop contractions and slow up your baby's arrival are controversial and can have side effects.

Dr. Howard Berk questions the success of drugs combined with bed rest. "I actually think that in the United States, modern obstetrical science has not decreased the number of premature babies going to the premature nursery by any drugs or any decision to go to bed. What we may be doing is taking a patient with regular, painless, uterine contractions but no change in her cervix, and saying, 'Well, you must be in labor,' when she isn't at all."

Berk believes that unless there is a change in the cervix, combined with painful contractions, it probably isn't premature labor. So, "Sending this woman to bed and giving her drugs is unnecessary," he says. On the other hand, if the cervix is starting to dilate and the uterus is contracting, "you can't really stop that birth from occurring," he explains. "What you can do is delay the event a little by going to bed, by raising your feet and relying on gravity, and by having a pessary (an instrument put into the vagina to support the uterus) inserted."

Not all cases of premature labor result in preterm birth. Although you may not really know exactly what triggered your early labor, if your contractions stop, your womb remains a healthy place for your baby to stay, no amniotic fluid has leaked, and your cervix is tightly closed, your pregnancy could proceed without further interruption. However, if your cervix softens, or effaces, and opens to more than four or five centimeters, early birth may be unavoidable. Rest assured that a very small percentage of babies are born prematurely, and with the advances in neonatology and obstetrical care, survival rates have increased dramatically. A regional network of perinatal care for premature infants, staffed by experts trained in the care of newborns at risk, is available to better your baby's chances of living happily ever after. Because operating these units is so expensive, not all hospitals offer this very special baby care with state-of-the-art maternal and fetal medicine. Hospitals fall into three categories as far as preemies' care is concerned: Level III, II, and I.

Level II hospitals can care for normal pregnancies and some high-risk cases. Sometimes, level II hospitals work closely with level IIIs on a consultation basis. If your hospital has a level I classification, it just isn't equipped to care for you on a long-term basis if you or your baby encounter special difficulties.

I Was Wondering . . .

I've read that exercise can help get me into shape for labor and delivery. Is it true? Should I start now?

Starting a brand-new exercise blitz late in pregnancy? Doing this in your twenty-eighth week is not a great idea. Making exercise a regular habit when you are pregnant is simply a wonderful move, but you should have started a bit earlier. In fact, if you are in your seventh month, you may be at the point in pregnancy when many doctors suggest that routines be cut back. Go for relaxation exercises or gentle stretches in preparation for birth at this point. Look at ways to curtail strenuous activities. Can you cut out working long shifts? Avoid standing on your feet or running yourself ragged in any way. In the meantime, moderate, low-impact, no-stress exercises can give you a sense of well-being. You just need to discuss your plans with your obstetrician before you start anything. Pregnancy, labor, and childbirth can make some pretty stiff demands on your body, so the more you prepare yourself physically, the better you will feel. The right kinds of exercise can help you with many of the common complaints of pregnancy: backaches, loss of bladder control, hemorrhoids, posture problems, and stiff muscles. Activity can increase your flexibility and make it easier for you to adjust your balance. That big belly can throw you off sometimes. Exercising regularly, but never to the point of exhaustion, can also decrease water retention and increase blood flow.

Get Help Right Away: Signs of Premature Labor

- Painful contractions every ten minutes or even more often.
- Cramps in your lower abdomen that remind you of menstrual pains.
- Pressure just above your pubic bone.
- Stomach pain.
- Backache at the bottom of your spinal cord. (This is a dull pain that's different from any other backaches you've had during pregnancy so far.)
- A change in your vaginal discharge. (You probably recognize the sticky, white leukorrhea by now. In premature labor, you could be leaking mucus that is watery or slightly bloody.)
- Blood stains on your underpants any time from the fifth to the ninth month.

Here are some pointers:

- Don't ever exercise until you are out of breath. The phrase, "no pain, no gain" does not apply to you now.
- Wear clothes that won't restrict your movements or make you sweat. Buy fabrics that let your skin "breathe."
- Avoid sports or any moves where there is danger of hurting your abdomen. Bike riding outside, skiing, water-skiing? Don't even think about it. In fact, skip anything that requires a lot of balance. Even aerobic dance routines may need to be adjusted to fit your state of life. Some jerky, bouncy numbers aren't great for your overstretched joints and ligaments. You don't want to try any muscular moves when you are lying on your back because you slow up the blood flow to the uterus and your unborn baby.
- Swim, walk, cycle on a stationary bicycle. Above all, keep it cool and think about sitting still, unless you are in a pool, on hot, overheated summer days.
- Stop immediately if you feel pain, get dizzy, faint, become breathless, or start bleeding.

My husband loves to play loud music. Is noise pollution harmful to our unborn baby?

You might want to ask him to turn down the volume. Exposure to noise, especially the kind that can be unexpected and uncontrollable, may affect your baby's health. Though amniotic fluid and the protection of your uterus do buffer the baby, harsh sounds can decrease fetal heart rates, according to a study conducted back in the 1940s. Finnish researchers also looked at the worrisome aspect of pregnancy and found that noise traveling through headphones didn't affect either mom or baby. Buy your mate some headphones so he can pump up the volume as high as he wants and remain in his own little world. Unborn babies do hear sounds, and certainly rock, twist, and turn to music, but you might want to think twice about what you are playing and how loud you set the volume.

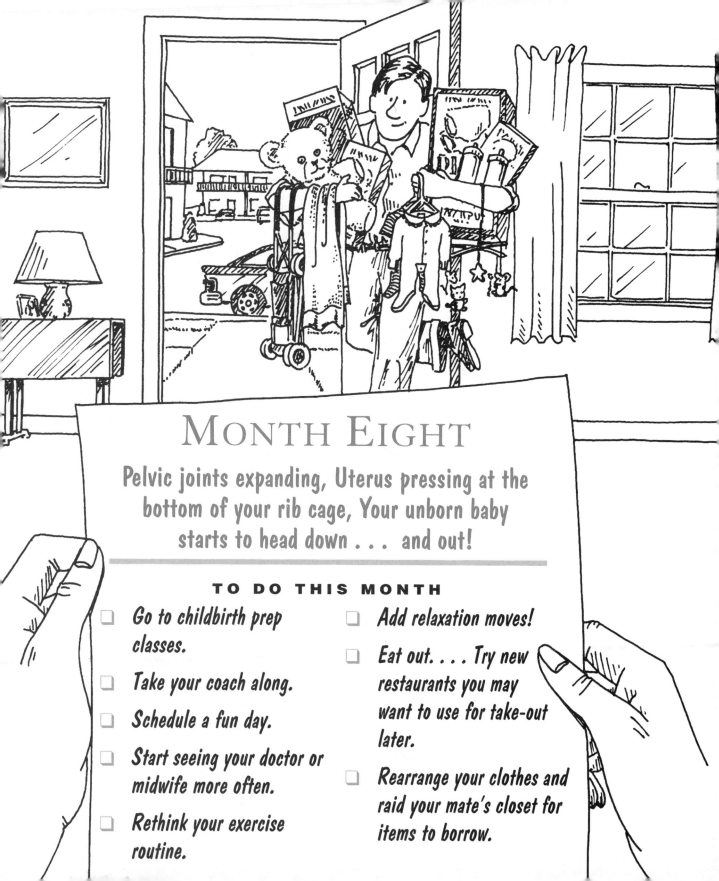

MONTH EIGHT

Pelvic joints expanding, Uterus pressing at the bottom of your rib cage, Your unborn baby starts to head down . . . and out!

TO DO THIS MONTH

☐ *Go to childbirth prep classes.*

☐ *Take your coach along.*

☐ *Schedule a fun day.*

☐ *Start seeing your doctor or midwife more often.*

☐ *Rethink your exercise routine.*

☐ *Add relaxation moves!*

☐ *Eat out. . . . Try new restaurants you may want to use for take-out later.*

☐ *Rearrange your clothes and raid your mate's closet for items to borrow.*

On the evening before my mother had her first child, my grandfather dropped her off at the entrance to a small hospital in Trenton, New Jersey, and wished her good luck. My father was off in the South Pacific serving his country during World War II, and she was in the early stages of labor with contractions far apart. Yet, even if my dad hadn't been thousands of miles away, he still wouldn't have been able to be with her as she gave birth to my older sister, Barbara. It just wasn't done back then. Husbands were supposed to pace nervously outside in the waiting room. Like almost all the other women giving birth in the 1940s in the United States, my mom would undergo one of life's most overwhelming experiences alone, intellectually unprepared, and emotionally scared to pieces. Her doctors and most others believed that even a little knowledge about birth was a dangerous thing for their patients.

Your birth experience will be very different from the lonely night my mother spent. When my son was born, I was hardly alone, and neither will you be if you arrange for your mate or someone else who knows you well to be with you and help you. Some childbirth classes call this special, supportive birthing partner a coach. *Coach* is a tame word for what's expected of your mate or how important having someone by your side is. Someone once said that the "presence of one husband during labor and delivery outweighs in value all the sedatives and medications in the world." My husband Bob held my hand for nearly twelve hours. I can still hear him dutifully calling out the practiced mantra he had picked up in our Lamaze childbirth classes. I was in labor with Zach, and Bob had learned his lessons well even though I turned out to be a C plus graduate. I'll admit it: I could hardly pay attention to anything but my convulsing belly.

"OK Maryann . . . now, here we go, fifteen seconds . . . (he'd say, trying to count down the contraction as if that would make me feel better) . . . thirty . . . forty-five . . . sixty . . . it's over . . . relax . . . relax."

Although I had been intellectually prepared by my Lamaze classes, I was still surprised by the intensity of the birth process. Knowing what to expect is going to help you, too. If you haven't begun taking childbirth preparation classes yet, don't delay another day. Sign up.

What Are You Feeling Emotionally

Uncertain and Fearful?

Lonnie Morris, a certified nurse-midwife and director of The Childbirth Center in Englewood, New Jersey, once said that the three biggest fears of expectant mothers under her care were:

1. *Will I have a normal baby?* Statistically speaking, yes, of course. Nature takes care of its own, Lonnie insists, and if you are eating enough of the right foods and taking good care of yourself, then your chances are even greater of having a perfectly normal baby. Even if your child is born with some kind of physical handicap, most conditions are treatable today, Lonnie points out.

2. *Can I get my baby out?* Hipbones have little to do with it. "I've seen little teeny women with teeny hipbones deliver great big babies—without episiotomies *(a small snip to widen the perineum before it tears during birth)*. Don't forget, only a small percentage of all babies need to be delivered by cesarean section," she says.

3. *Can I handle the responsibility of a new baby?* This is a fear you will have to work out on your own. Yes, of course, you can handle it, but you have to believe in yourself. This may be why second babies are almost always considered "better babies," according to Lonnie. "The mother is different. She's not afraid anymore. She forgets about time, about what she should be doing, about cobwebs on the ceiling—and follows the needs of the baby."

Unnerved and a Little Angry at Times?

As you become bigger, the stares, touches, reactions, and comments of outsiders can catch you off guard and make you wonder why people say or do such stupid things.

- "When are you due?" may become one of the most unnerving questions, especially if you have several weeks to go and you really don't care to share obstetrical details with total strangers. By the way, don't tell people exactly when you are due. Even if you mentioned the special date way

Soooo . . . Other Pregnant Women Have These Symptoms, Too:

- Tender, growing-even-bigger breasts that may leak sticky colostrum
- Lack of stamina
- Achy, swollen feet and puffy ankles, face, and hands
- Backaches
- Breathlessness, lightheadedness
- Frequent urination
- Insomnia
- Constipation, indigestion, heartburn, and stomach as well as intestinal gas
- Hemorrhoids
- Runny nose, stuffy sinuses
- Headaches
- Vaginal discharges
- Stretch marks and varicose veins
- Skin flareups and hair hassles
- Braxton-Hicks contractions
- Fetal movements

What to Buy Now for Your Baby

Clothes: You'll need five or six undershirts (both full-snap and half-shirt varieties), nightgowns with pull strings at the bottom, and nonflammable sleepers/rompers with covered feet. You will also need at least four pair of socks or booties (depending on your climate), one sweater or light jacket, two to four waterproof diaper covers, and one snowsuit (again, depending on the weather and when you deliver).

Bath items: You'll need a plastic bath tub or tub liner, baby soap, baby shampoo, baby lotion, two to four bath towels (preferably with hoods), or receiving blankets, three to four washcloths, sterile cotton balls and alcohol (to keep the umbilical cord clean until it heals).

Sleeptime items: You'll need a crib set (including a bumper pad, three to four fitted sheets, and two comforters), a bassinet sheet (if you are using a bassinet), waterproof crib liners, a light blanket or sheet for cover, a baby roll for propping baby to sleep on a particular side, and a music box or mobile.

Eating time items: You'll need four to six bottles (in both four- and eight-ounce sizes for water, breast milk, formula, or juice), a bottle brush, a bottle rack (for easy—and sterile—dishwasher cleaning), six to eight bibs and burping cloths, and, if nursing, at least two nursing bras, breast pads, and a breast pump (either manual or electric).

Changing time items: You'll need to stock your changing table with four or five undershirts or stretchies, petroleum jelly, baby wipes (alcohol free and hypoallergenic), a thermometer, a nasal aspirator, a pair of baby nail scissors, cotton balls and swabs, washcloths, diaper rash ointment, and, of course, hundreds of diapers!

back when, don't broadcast it repeatedly. Or try adding several weeks to the actual date when you tell others. Next month, this fictionalized delivery date will buy you peace and quiet as you draw closer to your rendezvous with a birthday. Everyone who wants to be the first to know will give you more time exactly when you need lots of rest during your ninth month. You won't have to answer the phone as much or return all those messages.

- "You look like you're carrying a . . . (boy? girl? twins?). New York physician Elizabeth Whelan, M.D. says that statistical analysis has proven that there is no way to tell, short of amniocentesis or X-ray, whether you are carrying a boy or girl, so don't fall victim to old wives' tales.

- "Reach out and touch someone" isn't just an advertising jingle at this point if you've found yourself fending off the touches of people wanting to pat your stomach. Remember, you have a right to your own space, so go ahead and follow your instinct as far as any unwanted gestures are concerned. Put yourself back in your prepregnant state. Would you want this particular person rubbing your stomach for good luck?

- You could also be made to feel as if you've come down with some dreadfully contagious disease because many people shy away from apparently pregnant women. Don't feel ashamed of your marvelous state of being.

- Jokes about your expectant state aren't always funny, so don't feel compelled to laugh or even behave courteously if you don't feel like it. "Soooo Big" is a game you may enjoy later with your baby or toddler, but when adults ogle you now and say, "Oh my, you are soooo big," you don't have to play along.

- Advice givers come out of the woodwork. Use what you like. Throw the rest away quickly, especially if it's negative.

- Others' expectations can make you nuts. Be yourself. Pay attention to your practitioner's advice, of course, but if working until the day before delivery is what makes you happy and you and your unborn baby appear to be healthy, then go for it. If you want to use this time as an excuse to sleep, eat, exercise, vacation, and have lots of fun, do it. If this is your first, in a few weeks, you'll need a babysitter to do some of the things you take for granted now.

Listen to This

In a 1965 edition of the medical journal *Practitioner*, a doctor by the name of J. D. Flew wrote, "Husbands should be in easy reach by telephone. . . . To me, the idea of the husband being present during the birth is repellant. It would put off my stroke and I would find it difficult to imagine any romance between this couple in the future." (Aren't you glad this guy isn't your doctor?) Dr. Joseph Rheingold, a crony of J. D. Flew, concurred in his book, *The Fear of Being a Woman*, and wrote, "Mature women do not wish their husbands to attend the delivery."

My how times have changed for the better. Go to class together if you can. As Elisabeth Bing, well-known authority in childbirth education, has said, "Pregnancy can be the first real challenge a couple faces together in marriage. Talking about it, learning about pregnancy and birth can help. In each class, a few expectant fathers admit that they have been 'dragged' over."

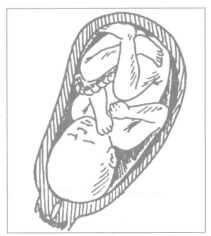

At 32 weeks, the head is now more in proportion to the body.

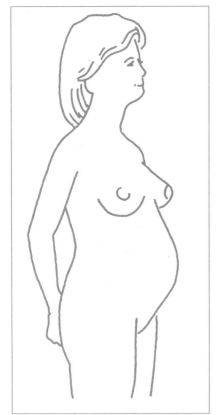

Weight gain should start to slow down during this month.

Oh Baby . . . Inside Secrets

- Near the end of this month, your unborn baby could be as long as sixteen and one-half to eighteen inches long and could weigh five pounds.
- Proportionally, the little body now looks like the head belongs. Fetal heads are disproportionly large for the size of those developing bodies up until the eighth month.
- Stockpiling all the immunities, your baby spends some time and energy this month borrowing all that he or she can from you. The natural immunities it has taken you years to build will help your baby stay healthy during those first few months after birth.
- Fatter and bigger, your child doesn't have as much kicking, twisting, or turning room inside the uterus. What used to feel like swooping or swimming inside has now turned into real jabbing and pushing. Stay tuned to those maneuvers now. If you detect less than ten a day, let your doctor know right away. However, as the baby finds less space for physical fun, quiet times may last longer.
- Brain cells are just expanding wildly this month and will continue this fast-paced course steadily now. Talk to your baby. Play music. Have your husband or any siblings introduce themselves. These familiar voices and sounds can be heard inside.
- Chances of survival outside your body now are marvelous. (If you've been worried about premature labor or have been placed in a high-risk category for any reason, you can feel a bit more comfortable about your body as a baby-making vehicle. Relax . . . you've almost made it to the finish line.)
- Gradually shifting to the same position in which 95 percent of all babies are born, your fetus starts to head down, pushing into your pubic area upside down. This move to what is known as the *vertex position* is especially predictable for first births. If your doctor happens to mention that your baby's bottom seems to be descending into your pelvis, as opposed to his or her head, she may be concerned about a *breech birth*, in which the buttocks or feet emerge first.

Choosing a Pediatrician

Ask your practitioner to recommend baby doctors. Friends, family members, and your regular family doctor can also be good sources of great baby doctors. You will also want to check your insurance plan or health maintenance organization for listing of pediatric practices included in your regular coverage. Don't wait until after your baby arrives to do this sort of homework. A pediatrician can be part of your team when you deliver the baby, checking on your newborn and answering any questions you may have as a brand-new mom. In fact, find out if the doctors on your list have visiting privileges at the hospital or birthing center where you are scheduled for birth.

Phone first and jot down general impressions. Is the receptionist rude? Do you sense frustration or ridicule in the doctor's voice? You want a professional who will take you as well as your baby's needs seriously. Ask yourself if he or she is a person who respects women, especially new mothers in crises? You don't want to anticipate the worst of your first months of parenting, but you do want to know that your child's doctor will not dismiss your fears or concerns as unfounded. When you get a positive feeling from the staff, set up an appointment to interview the pediatrician. This person will be caring for your child from birth up to age sixteen. You are interviewing someone for a very important job and not just any name on your list will do. Here are some questions you may want to ask when you meet face to face:

- What do you find most fulfilling about working with youngsters?
- What kind of regular office policies do you practice? (For instance, are all sick kids sequestered in the same waiting room? Contagious illnesses can spread quickly if this is the case.)
- What is your philosophy regarding parents? Are you a parent yourself?
- Do you have any rules or regulations regarding emergencies?
- What is the average waiting time for your regular office visits?
- Are there any special hours during which you take informational telephone calls from parents?
- Will insurance cover all, if not most, of your fees and special requests?

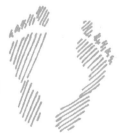

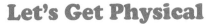

Let's Get Physical
You're Normal If . . .

- Your pelvic joints hurt. The pelvis has to stretch for your baby to have room to be born; and in this last trimester, your joints, ligaments, and bones may actually feel sore. The joints loosen up in a rather extraordinary way because of both the hormonal and the physical changes taking place. This remarkable ability is one of the reasons why some very small women are able to give birth to rather large babies. Early in pregnancy, the size of your pelvic joints isn't really a good indication of whether you will be able to deliver vaginally.

- Clumsy could be your middle name now, especially when you walk or try to run. You feel downright bulky, but don't always realize how out of balance you really are. In your mind, you may still have that prepregnant body. When I was eight months pregnant, I remember thinking that I could run across the street to beat a traffic light and catch a train. Not only did I fail to make allowances for my loosening pelvic joints but the shift in my body's balance because I was carrying at least thirty extra pounds right out front was dramatic. I fell forward and almost gave the crossing guard a heart attack. I was fine. My baby was fine. I missed my train, but decided to take it slow from that point on. Don't be hard on yourself emotionally if you start to turn into one of those pregnant ladies who waddles slightly when she walks.

- Your underpants could end up wet when you laugh or sneeze. Not only can all this increased pressure on your bladder send you to the bathroom a zillion times each day and into the night, but also sudden quick movements like a laugh or sneeze can make it hard for you to control your urine. This is called *stress incontinence* and is due to the progesterone in your body causing relaxation of the bladder and the sphincter. If you suspect that you are leaking more than urine and the drips could be amniotic fluid, call your doctor and explain your worry right away.

- Hemorrhoids could become a real pain. The pressure of your baby's head in your pelvic cavity can cause swollen veins around your anus. If you've been having bouts of constipation during your pregnancy, this hemorrhoidal condition can become a constant, itchy, painful, irksome problem. Whenever you strain to empty your bowels, the situation can make you want to scream. Hemorrhoids

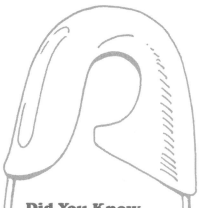

can even bleed. Don't be shy about asking your doctor to recommend help. Put an ice pack against the hemorrhoids. Don't stand in any situation where a seat is possible. (More tips on helping ease hemorrhoid pain are found in Month Four.)

- Your breathlessness may have gotten worse. Your uterus might be pressing on the bottom of your rib cage right up on your diaphragm, making you uncomfortable and breathless. Let's face it, your lungs are crowded. Your need to breathe slowly and deeply isn't affecting your baby's growth—unless you are trying to run a marathon. If you are carrying low, breathlessness isn't such a discomfort. Try not to slouch. When you stand or sit up straight, you get more air into your lungs. Prop a pillow up behind you in bed if getting to sleep is a problem.

- Friends say you look a little puffy. This mild swelling in your face, around your eyes, lips, and in your hands and lower limbs is quite common and might be in your lower legs, ankles, and feet. Known as *edema*, it's normal, and you could even have as much as thirteen extra pints of fluid during these last weeks. There's no need to cut down your salt intake, however. Rest. Nap every day. Watch for signs of extreme and sudden swelling, of course.

- You could have a significantly dark line running down your abdomen (the *linea nigro*).

- The veins in your breasts are more prominent.

- You've put on lots of your pregnant pounds by now. Although the obstetrical rule of thumb is for your weight gain to start slowing down now, that doesn't always happen. Your womb is still expanding, your placenta is still working its marvelous wonders, your blood volume is up, your baby is putting on pounds, and your overall body fat composition has changed for good reasons. Fat may be concentrated on your hips, breasts, and thighs, and these stores act like nutritional reserve. After delivery, the extra fat helps you become a better breastfeeder. (Even if you aren't going to breastfeed, the fat does tend to drop off in the postpartum period.) Almost all of your baby's weight gain takes place during the last trimester, so please don't limit yourself or try to diet. Are you getting 2,600 calories each day? If not, eat up. If so, pat yourself on the back and don't feel guilty about gaining now.

Did You Know . . .

The size of your pelvic joints isn't really a good indication of whether or not your baby will make an easy appearance?

Ninety-five percent of all babies are born head-down, or *vertex* position?

You've probably gained about 35 percent of your pregnant weight by now?

Lamaze birthing ideas are based on a Russian researcher's discovery?

Ignorance about labor and delivery can actually make it hurt more?

Lots of expectant couples who can't decide on baby names are using the Internet to gather ideas?

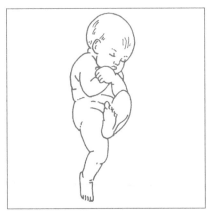

Incomplete (footling) breech.

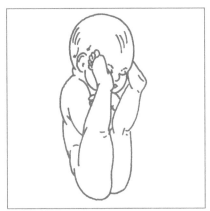

Frank breech.

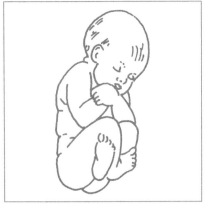

Complete (full) breech.

A Breech Birth?

If your practitioner brings up the question of a breech, or buttocks-first, birth during one of your routine office visits during the last trimester, it's because she or he has felt the hard head of your unborn baby up near your ribs. You may have detected feet or a little bottom down below closer to your pelvis. This unwieldy positioning can definitely shift and change in the next few weeks, and your practitioner may even try to turn the baby using a technique known as *external cephalic version*. Your practitioner may be concerned because a baby in this breech position is more difficult to deliver and cesarean sections are more likely to ease your baby safely out. Only 3 to 4 percent of babies are born buttocks first. This incidence goes up for premature births. Other factors, such as excessive amniotic fluid, an abnormal uterus, the location of the placenta, and a history of multiple births, add to the chances of breech positioning. There are actually three classifications of breech: frank, complete, and incomplete. In *frank breech*, your baby shows up bottom first with his or her legs tucked up close to the chest. The lowest number of breech complications are associated with frank. Theoretically with incomplete, as your cervix dilates in labor and the baby begins the trip down the birth canal, one or both legs will drop down and will arrive before the rest of the body. You may hear someone describe this as a *single or double footling breech birth*. If your baby insists on arriving in what is called a *complete breech*, his bottom is first, but legs and arms are crossed in front of his little body. Another unusual position your practitioner may notice during routine physical exams of your abdomen, also known as palpations, is the *transverse position*, in which the baby is sideways in your womb.

In Your Doctor's Bag of Tools, Tests & Requests

You will be trudging into your practitioner's office more often now, probably every two weeks this month and then weekly.

Tests for high blood pressure, blood sugar levels, and protein in your urine specimen continue. You'll be watched for any extreme swelling in your hands, feet, or face. Using your own baseline pressure as a gauge, if your blood pressure shoots up more than thirty points in the upper range or fifteen points in the lower number, this is a sign of preeclampsia, sometimes called *toxemia*, or *pregnancy-induced hypertension*. By now, you've grown accustomed to the cuff, stethoscope, or electronic measurement of your blood pressure.

Checks for a substance called *albumin* in your urine sample are also routine by now, another potential sign of toxemia. Too much albumin indicates trouble. If your level is too high, a special test may be ordered. If your practitioner schedules you for what is called a glucose tolerance test (GTT), blood samples are taken before and after you are given a special glucose drink. The test measures your body's ability to handle sugar in the bloodstream and can indicate women who may be more likely to have diabetic conditions during their pregnancies. Statistics vary on the number of pregnant women who do end up with gestational diabetes, but this test is often given sometime between the twenty-fourth and twenty-eighth week. If you have shown signs of sugar in your urine earlier or were placed in a high-risk category because of obesity or prior complications in pregnancy, you may already be familiar with the GTT routine. Most blood sugar problems disappear after pregnancy; and because practitioners are now so skilled at recognizing and preparing for diabetes during pregnancy, most pregnancies proceed without problems. Relax.

Meanwhile, a little extra sugar in your urine isn't out of the ordinary during pregnancy; but if your levels are persistently high, the doctor may be worried about complications from gestational diabetes.

I Was Wondering . . .

Because we live about forty minutes away from the hospital where I expect to deliver my baby, I'm worried about getting there in time. This is our first. Is it too soon to start practicing the trip?

No, it's not too soon to make a practice run, even though your chances of not making it to the hospital for delivery on time are low. Most first births don't happen instantaneously. Yet, go ahead and practice at a time when you can map out the best streets and roads to take. Later on, when you are in labor, timing contractions, and trying to stay calm, you'll be glad you know the least stressful route. Figure out which hospital or clinic door you are supposed to enter and ask about filling out any preliminary paperwork beforehand. If you are scheduled to give birth in a big city hospital, be aware of what rush hour traffic congestion will add to your trip's length. Plan ahead. Fill the gas tank of your car and keep it filled. Or, set aside cash for taxis or a car service. Don't forget money for toll roads or bridges if you are going by private car. Don't worry excessively about arriving in time for the birth. The average first labor lasts from twelve to fourteen hours and the longest part comes first. Did you know that some experts believe that a labor should last from eleven to fifteen hours in order for your skin to stretch and your baby to move down the birth canal? Although your forty-minute drive seems to be adding anxiety to your anticipation now, the trip may actually keep your mind occupied especially if you have done your advance homework and know exactly where you are going and what to expect when you arrive.

A new friend from childbirth class, who is also eight months pregnant, just had a special test performed because she was worried about a lack of fetal movement. I think it was called a nonstress or anti-stress test. Can you tell me more about this?

To measure fetal heart rate, your doctor can use at least two tests before labor begins: the nonstress test and the contraction stress test, according to the American College of Obstetricians and Gynecologists (ACOG). Both rely on the fetal heart monitor. Your new friend probably had a belt strapped around her abdomen. A *nonstress test* would measure the heart rate in response to the baby's own movement. Ordinarily the heart beat speeds up during any kind of activity, even a whoosh or a push by the baby. Any change is considered a good indication of things proceeding along without complications. Your pregnant friend may have been lying on a bed or up on an examining table during the procedure for about twenty minutes. She could have been asked to press a button every time she felt the baby move. The beats are recorded on a paper and tend to be very reassuring for everyone, especially a worried expectant mom.

If the test was a *contraction stress test* (CST), her practitioner may have been concerned about how the baby would react during labor. When your uterus contracts, blood flow to the placenta and to the baby slows down temporarily so there may be some concern about how effective the placenta is working. If the fetal heart falls with contractions, this is an indication to consider immediate delivery. Blood flow to the placenta decreases with contractions. If the baby cannot maintain a good heart rate during this time, then he or she may be in some degree of distress. During a contraction, the baby's heart, lungs, and systems should be able to survive without any changes for that forty-second length. To initiate mild contractions, your friend may have been given *oxytocin*, a drug to induce laborlike contractions. This procedure can take up to two hours, according to ACOG. Ordinarily a doctor won't order this unless the nonstress test produces unsatisfactory results. Don't worry about premature labor being induced during the test. Risk is minimal because minimal amounts of oxytocin are used.

If a *biophysical profile* was performed, this just means that the technician used the data to get a clearer picture not only of the fetal heart rate but also of the baby's muscle tone, body movement, and the amniotic fluid in the womb. Adding this step to the testing regimen may have added another half-hour to your friend's experience. Lots of good information can be picked up during a biophysical profile. For instance, although the baby isn't really breathing yet, what experts look for are signs of the little chest moving in and out. Each item in a biophysical profile is scored, and if the number obtained is between eight and ten, then everything is within normal range. Too low a number is cause for concern and the test may be redone to get a better picture of what's happening. A score of two or less is considered an obstetrical emergency calling for immediate intervention.

Will I be overwhelmed by the pain of labor?

Probably not, because you will be prepared. First of all, you are reading this book. You are (or already have) taken classes, too. Your attitude is also going to make a tremendous difference. There is just no way to predict the intensity of your labor and delivery. After my

---

**Doctor's Note:
To Calm Fears
of Labor**

An epidural can be used early in labor to help a woman gain control of her fears and the pain. Of course, the best time to insert the epidural is when she has reached four centimeters, but if I have a patient who is extremely worried and can't calm her fears, I'll use it sooner. By using pitocin and a fetal monitor in conjunction with this early epidural, I can even talk the patient through the pushing stage of delivery and she doesn't have to feel anything. *(Read more about epidurals on page 220.)*
—Howard Berk, M.D.

Baby Shower Games

Baby showers can be a lot more fun when you play silly games. Seriously, sometimes the sillier the game, the more fun you'll have. Here are just a few activities suggested by Katina Z. Jones, author of *The Everything Get Ready for Baby Book*:

- Baby naming: With a timer in hand, ask the guests to write down as many girl and boy names as they can in one minute. Whoever comes up with the most names wins. Make the game more challenging by limiting names to those beginning with a specific letter.

- Total recall: Place a dozen baby-related items on a tray, and then let the guests see the items for thirty to forty-five seconds. Cover the tray; whoever remembers and writes down the most items wins a prize.

- So big: How big is the mom-to-be's belly? If you were to wrap toilet paper around her, how many squares do you think it would take?

- Mystery food: Put twelve baby-food jars—labels hidden—on a tray, and place the tray in the middle of a table for fifteen minutes. Use more trays for larger groups. Whoever can identify all or most of the mystery foods wins a prize.

- Pin the diaper on the baby: No, not the real baby—just a large picture of a baby. Mount the picture on a piece of cardboard, and then give each guest a picture of a diaper with tape on the back. See how close to the target area they can pin the diaper—while blindfolded, of course.

- Guess how many: Put as many pieces of candy into a large baby bottle as you can; whoever guesses the right amount wins the candy as a prize.

- Name that tune: Using a spoon or similar object, play lullabies and other well-known baby songs by tapping the spoon on an oatmeal container. Whoever can guess the most songs wins.

- Special day: Whoever's birthday is closest to the baby's due date wins a prize.

first birth, still somewhat shocked by how much hard work was demanded of me, I turned to my obstetrician and asked, "Why didn't you tell me?" He replied, "Because every woman's experience is different. If I told you it was going to hurt like h___, I could have frightened you without cause."

Your pain, if you have any, is going to be manageable because you'll be in the hands of a professional you know and trust and you will have a coach or partner who is well prepared to take care of you when you are most vulnerable. You also have the wonders of modern medical pain relief available to you at important points in your progress. Believe me, any so-called agonies of your birth experience are not going to rival those classic descriptions in literature. For instance, if you are worried about having the kind of birth described in Dostoyevsky's *Anna Karenina*, don't. "Flushed . . . agonized . . . the terrible screams followed each other until they seemed to reach the utmost limit of horror." Or perhaps the depiction of birth in *Tom Jones* has you in its grip. "I became a mother by the man I scored, hated and detested. I went through all the agonies and miseries of lying in . . . in a desert or rather, indeed, a scene of riot and revel, without a friend, without a companion, which often alleviate and perhaps sometimes more than compensate the sufferings of our sex at that time." See there . . . even Mrs. Fitzpatrick realized that having the right help could and should have made the difference. In the meantime, keep reading, don't stop asking questions and gathering birth stories. Examples of women who breeze through birth are just as plentiful as those who don't ever want to remember what it felt like. Make up your own mind that you will be able to manage anything that comes your way . . . one step at a time.

My husband and I have been having a continuing "discussion" about baby names. Do you have any suggestions for where to find good ideas?

Naming a baby can be fun as well as frustratingly difficult. Try not to approach the process with your mind set about any particular name or pet peeve about something your mate has in mind.

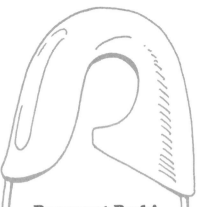

Pregnant Perk!

Look at Time as Your Life

When you stop trying to spend, save, or invest your time, you'll feel less burdened by stress. Of course, your time is important, especially now with only a few weeks to go before your due date, but by looking at it from a rushed, mercenary point, you may be missing out on so much that is truly enjoyable. You'll never be at this point in your baby-making career again. Find a way to enjoy your time.

Consider the names on your family trees. Jot down both of your favorites. Browse through some of the great books available, which can offer tips on combining first and last names so the syllables fall into perfect sync and to avoid unfortunate initials. Along with all the great books of baby names on store shelves, you will find a veritable wealth of advice and ideas by searching the Internet. Even if you don't have your own computer connection at home, this quest for the perfect name may be something you want to do at the public library or anywhere you can find access to a computer on the World Wide Web. Using the Yahoo search engine, I was impressed by what is available and by expectant couples who were asking for input from the kindness of strangers about what to name their babies. I encountered a contest posted. Researchers at one site had combed through Social Security Administration records back to 1930 to come up with names ranked both in popularity from year to year as well as alphabetical order. Biblical names, Irish names, Indian, Hindu, Sikh names, as well as hints for combining words. The Utah Baby Namer listed odd names unique to Utah Mormon culture. One of my favorite Web sites was the Baby Name Finder (http://bnf.parentsoup.com) and by tapping in my own name, I found out that Maryann is a three-syllable girl's name of Hebrew/Greek origin meaning, "The perfect one; bitter; with sorrow; grace." I also learned that 33 percent of people with my name spell it the same way I do. Zachary, my son, turns out to have been named at the beginning of a trend. Zach is a newcomer to the top fifty most popular boy's names in the United States, but wasn't even noticeable until the 1980s. Meanwhile, my daughter's name, Maggie, a nickname for Margaret, which is what we put on her official birth certificate, is a name that has been consistently popular for generations. I laughed when I saw that Margaret is a good choice for insecure parents because of the amazing number of possible nicknames. This is exactly what we were thinking when we debated what she might want to be called at age seventeen! We still call her Maggie, just as we did the day she was born.

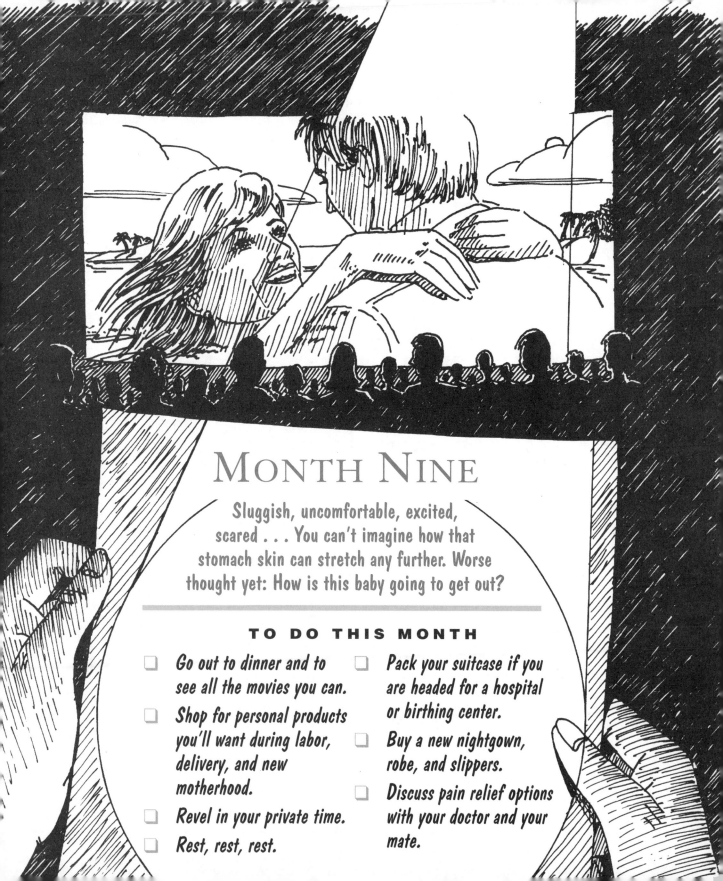

MONTH NINE

Sluggish, uncomfortable, excited, scared . . . You can't imagine how that stomach skin can stretch any further. Worse thought yet: How is this baby going to get out?

TO DO THIS MONTH

- ☐ Go out to dinner and to see all the movies you can.
- ☐ Shop for personal products you'll want during labor, delivery, and new motherhood.
- ☐ Revel in your private time.
- ☐ Rest, rest, rest.
- ☐ Pack your suitcase if you are headed for a hospital or birthing center.
- ☐ Buy a new nightgown, robe, and slippers.
- ☐ Discuss pain relief options with your doctor and your mate.

Four weeks to go. Sometimes when you look at yourself in the shower or catch a glance in a department store mirror, you can't imagine that this is you. That old familiar body is nowhere in sight, and yet, in your mind's eye, you may still be the same old you inside. At a fancy restaurant with my husband and some friends near the end of my first pregnancy, I remember rising from the table before dessert was served so I could make another trip to the bathroom. Looking for the best route through the tables and past the dessert cart, I made a quick decision based on the size and space my body had once been. Big mistake! Squeezing between a chair and the cart loaded with luscious-looking sweets and treats, I caught my stomach on the corner and almost took the cart with me to the ladies' room door.

What Are You Feeling Emotionally?

Tired of Being Pregnant?

If you are physically active, then this last month can be a trial. You simply can't move as easily as you were able to do eight months ago. With thoughts focused on the birth ahead of you and your attention continually on those signs, symptoms, and twitches that might indicate impending labor, you may feel that time is a real drag. While some of the unwelcome physical symptoms (breathlessness, heartburn, indigestion) may start to lessen as the baby drops down into your pelvis, the heavy load in your lower abdomen can make you frustrated about moving at all. What was new, interesting, fascinating, or even marvelous about being pregnant can become old by now. Even your fear of the unknown may seem to pale now compared to your urge to get over being pregnant, meet your baby, and get on with your life. Relax, this may feel like the longest month of your life, but when you look back later, you may see it as the quiet before the whirlwind of new motherhood.

Annoyed?

Little things can ratchet up your frustration level easily. Even a trip to the bathroom, which you may be doing zillions of times a day and into the night, can take a toll. You can't bend down to tie your own shoes without twisting yourself around and over that growing belly. Constant comments of friends as well as strangers can try your patience. Exactly how many times must you answer the questions, "How are you?" "When are you due?" Your dependency on others can also be annoying. I hated being conspicuous and when people said, "Let me help you with that . . . " I didn't want to be polite.

Worried?

Your fears can take on frightening proportions this month if you let them. Don't keep them to yourself. Share your thoughts. Even wild-eyed worries really do have solutions when you ask the right person. Speak up.

Excited and Happy?

By reaching this stage of your baby-making marathon, you must give yourself the credit you deserve. Think back to how you felt when you first realized that your body was cooperating and you were pregnant. Treat yourself to an outing, an outfit, a meal, or just time off for such good biological behavior. Steal an entire day from what may be a busy schedule and create a happy memory of this ninth month odyssey.

Compelled to Clean and Decorate?

Known as the *nesting instinct*, this drive to straighten up your house, clean out closets, and decorate the baby's space isn't universal, but fairly common. In their ninth months, some women have been known to iron, scrub, wash curtains, empty drawers, rearrange furniture (with help, of course), and simply notice what's missing from their surroundings. I think that's when I started becoming more interested in decorating magazines. However, if this urge to clean and clear out doesn't strike you, don't berate yourself. An overweening nesting instinct can also send you to the hospital if you aren't careful to slow down and take it easy.

Soooo . . . Other Pregnant Women Have These Symptoms, Too:

- Tender, growing-even-bigger breasts that may leak sticky colostrum
- Lack of stamina
- Achy, swollen feet and puffy ankles, face, and hands
- Backaches
- Breathlessness, lightheadedness
- Frequent urination
- Insomnia
- Constipation, indigestion, heartburn, and stomach as well as intestinal gas
- Hemorrhoids
- Runny nose, stuffy sinuses
- Headaches
- Vaginal discharges
- Stretch marks and varicose veins
- Skin flareups and hair hassles
- Braxton-Hicks contractions
- Fetal movements

Preparing a Sibling

The arrival of a new sibling can be a joyous occasion for a young child. But it is not without its challenges, since some children would prefer that they be the apple of Mom's (or Dad's) eye. The hardest part for children to understand, according to Katina Z. Jones, author of *The Everything Get Ready for Baby Book*, is not necessarily that there's a new baby coming but rather why: "Why do you need to have another baby, Mommy? Aren't I good enough for you? Why do I have to share my room with the baby? Why do I have to give the baby my old clothes and toys?"

Here are ways to make the transition smoother:

- Make the pregnancy seem real from the start. Use age-related books to teach your child about the intricate process of growing a baby. Talk about the story of your child's birth, too. Nothing helps a sibling-to-be understand better than the details about the who, what, when, where, and how of his or her own birth.
- Allow your child hands on experience feeling the baby move.
- If possible, take your child with you to the doctor's office.
- Encourage your child to ask questions and try to answer them as best you can.
- Involve your child in preparing the "nest."
- Bring out your child's baby scrapbook if you have kept one updated.
- Tell your child what will happen at the hospital or birthing center and be honest about the new baby.
- Pack a special present for your child in your hospital bag, and give it to him or her when presenting the new baby.
- Be firm and direct about your child's feelings and the way they are acted out. Don't try to talk a child out of legitimate emotions. Feeling negative or left out are to be expected. However, hitting or abusing the new baby is definitely unacceptable.
- Set and keep a "special" time together.

Oh Baby . . . Inside Secrets Now

- Your baby is gaining up to one ounce a day now, could weigh as much as five to six pounds and be more than eighteen inches long. By week 40, he or she may be up to or over the seven and one-half pound mark and twenty inches in length.
- Fat deposits beneath the skin make the baby look plumper.
- Teeny, but softly sharpened, nails have grown to the tips of fingers and toes and could be the cause of little scratch marks you'll notice on your baby's skin at birth.
- If it's a boy, the testicles have descended and are now apparent in ultrasound images.
- Arms and legs are in a flexed position.
- Lungs are fully mature and ready to operate in the outside world.
- A dark, tarlike substance called *meconium* is in your baby's intestines and will become the contents of his or her first bowel movement.
- The lanugo, or downy hair, covering the body is disappearing along with the vernix, or cheesy protective coating. A bit of vernix may remain behind in the cracks and crevices of skin folds.
- Movement will slow down as you get closer to your due date, but a baby in trouble will also try to conserve energy by staying too quiet. When you wake up in the morning and just before you go to bed, take a half hour to sit still and count the number of kicks you feel inside. More than five or six should be enough to make you rest easier mentally that all is safe inside your private little world. Even ten moves a day are fine.

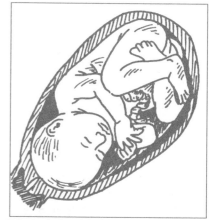

At the beginning of the 9th month, hair might have grown as much as two inches, and skin takes a pinkish hue.

Let's Get Physical

- Your lower abdomen feels heavy as the baby drops down headfirst to get ready for delivery.
- No matter how much weight you may have gained, relax. A lot of it will disappear soon. Remember . . . those extra pounds break down like this: 38 percent is baby; 22 percent is blood and fluid; 20 percent is pure womb, breasts,

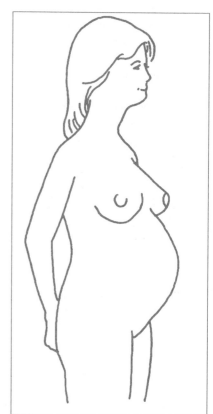

Good posture is critical as the position of the womb alters your usual weight distribution.

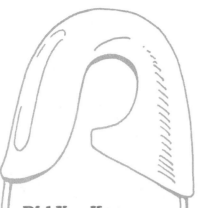

Did You Know . . .

The *nesting instinct* is not an imaginary, birdlike phenomenon. If you start cleaning or redecorating now, you've got it!

A snack or glass of juice can make your blood sugar rise and get your baby up and moving about?

Your vagina looks purple because it's stretched and engorged with blood?

The hardest phase of labor is the shortest?

Forceps were invented by a pair of secretive English brothers back in 1588?

Average babies move less now and are down from the 500 flips, kicks, and turns in Week 32 to a mere 280?

buttocks, and your legs; 11 percent is amniotic fluid; and 9 percent is the placenta.

- Your cervix is softening and getting ready to dilate, or open, to let your baby out and your vagina has stretched, too. Not only has the vagina increased in length, but because the veins are engorged with blood, it could look a bit purplish. You may also have noticed an increase in vaginal discharge, which is being caused by secretions from your cervix.
- Concentrate on good posture now because your baby is throwing your balance off more than ever before. Backaches can be everyday affairs. Don't lie flat on your back. Getting into such a prone position can take your breath away or even make you feel sick to your stomach.
- Keep on moisturizing any stretch marks on your breasts or expanding belly. Most of the time, these lines lighten and almost disappear after birth, but if they are really worrying you, ask your doctor about remedies. Some reports indicate that a safe pulsed eye laser can erase the unsightly reminders of your skin's elasticity.
- Slow down and relax because, in theory, the hormones released in your body when you are stressed can cause early contractions.
- Put your feet up whenever you can now. Sit still or, if it's summertime, soak in a swimming pool. An indoor pool is also nice. Almost all expectant moms have fluid, which shows up in the ankles, feet, and lower legs during this last month. You can cut down on this edema by resting with your legs elevated as often as possible. One report indicated that a dip in a shoulder-deep pool can also offer effective relief. No pool in sight? Fill your bathtub with cool water and slip in. While taking a bath in the last weeks of pregnancy used to be prohibited because of fear of infection from dirty bath water, this warning is no longer considered appropriate. Your baby is well protected until the mucus plug is eliminated or the amniotic sac ruptures.

Practical Pointers

It's not too soon to get organized for labor, delivery, and those days of brand-new motherhood. You may want to stockpile basic food items and plan for easy meals now when you have two hands to prepare and your thinking is clear. After your baby is born, you will be preoccupied. Believe me, you will be absolutely ecstatic and relieved about any meals you have prepared ahead. If you have a freezer, use it. You might even want to pick up take-out menus from restaurants in your area that deliver. Put them in a handy kitchen drawer.

Get your suitcase out and open it in your bedroom. Some hospital-based childbirth classes offer a helpful list of things to pack for both labor and recovery.

What to Pack for Labor

- *Loose fitting T-shirt or nightgown.* Hospital gowns aren't always comfortable and your own familiar shirt or nightie could make you feel like you've brought a piece of home to a strange place. You are going to sweat buckets, so keep this factor prominently in your mind.
- *Socks* to keep your feet warm.
- *Deodorant and talcum powder* to make you feel fresher and to dust lightly on your back before your coach gives you a massage.
- *Cosmetic bag packed with toothpaste, toothbrush, and lip balm.*
- *Gadgets to get you through labor.* Hot water bottles for backaches, tennis balls for your coach to apply pressure, a small natural sponge to dip in cool water for sucking, a poster of a beautiful vacation spot to put on the wall, your own favorite pillow, or anything your instructor recommends to help you through the hours of contractions.
- *Snacks and drinks.* You may not be allowed or even up for food and nourishment once your labor gets underway, but your coach could use some fortification for the long haul.
- *Books, magazines, things to read.*

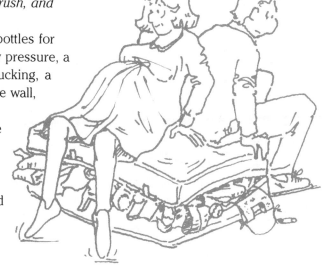

- *Stereo headphones* to listen to your favorite tapes or CDs and drown out other hospital or birthing center noises.
- *Phone numbers* of important people you will want to call, as well as change for the pay telephone or your phone card credit number.
- *A celebration kit.* Champagne or sparkling cider to toast your success when you are in the recovery room.
- *A watch or clock* with a second hand that is easy to see so you can time contractions.
- *Your camera* to record the birth. Some couples bring along video cameras to capture everything on tape for posterity. Not all hospitals allow videotapings, however.

What to Pack for after the Birth

Don't put these items in your labor pile. Even if you are going to use one suitcase, put these items in separately because you'll want to have them after you have delivered your baby and are in your own room or getting ready to go home. Use your creativity. Consider your comfort. Add things you know you will want to have handy.

- *Two to three machine-washable, cotton nightgowns* with front openings.

    Even though you don't think you'll be staying long, you want to be ready for an emergency. Extra nighties are not going to take up that much space in your suitcase. Buttons or snaps down the front will make it easier for you to open and close your gown to ease your baby in and out if you are planning to breastfeed. Cotton won't make you sweat.
- *A comfortable bathrobe*

    For wandering the hallways and greeting visitors
- *Comfy slippers*

    For taking walks
- *Brush, comb, shampoo, hairdryer*

    You'll definitely want to wash and fix your hair.
- *Two boxes of sanitary pads*

    You may be dealing with a lot of bloody discharge, called *lochia,* for several weeks after the birth and tampons are not recommended. Stock up on pads now and put some in your suitcase. Try to find the longest pads available.

- *Breast pads*
  To slip inside your bra for leaky nipples if you plan on breastfeeding.
- *Ointment or cream for sore breasts*
  Ask your doctor or midwife for recommendations. I used vitamin E oil when I was nursing for the first few weeks.
- *Two to three nursing bras* if you plan to nurse or regular ones (the same size you've been wearing now in the third trimester) if you have opted for bottle-feeding.
- *Six pairs of underpants*
  Pack a pile and make them cotton. You may go through quite a few in the first days of new motherhood.
- *An outfit for going home*
  Think comfortable first and not high-fashion, necessarily. Tight-fitting jeans won't work.
- *An outfit for the baby*, which might include a stretch suit or little nightie, undershirt, sweater, hat, receiving blanket, or warmer outerwear if you are delivering in winter in a cold climate. Don't forget diapers. Some hospitals have going-away gift packages full of free samples for new mothers and babies, but you shouldn't count on it. Buy one box of the very smallest size newborn diapers even though you think you are having the biggest baby in the world.
- *Infant car seat.*
  Most hospitals won't let you take the baby home without one.

In Your Doctor's Bag of Tools and Tests

An Arsenal of Pain Relief Options

Predicting how painful your labor will be is impossible. Even if this is a second or third pregnancy, your experience could be different each time. Sit down with your practitioner and review all your options

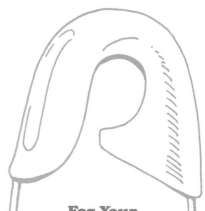

For Your Information

In a study conducted by Dr. Eliahu Sadovsky at Hadassah University Hospital in Jerusalem, a tally of average daily fetal movements was taken for 127 pregnant women who later delivered normally. From Week 20 on, babies moved about 200 times a day, and this activity escalated until Week 32, when they reached a point of 500 kicks, flips, and turns each day. After that point, the movements dropped to about 280 times daily. If you notice a real slowdown in activity, let your doctor know right away. Try eating a snack or drinking a glass of juice to make your blood sugar rise to see if the increase will stimulate your baby. Let your practitioner know when or if you feel that something is not quite right.

for pain relief. Even if you have already discussed this topic, bring it up again now. Get a full professional description of the differences between each type of pain medication available, including pros, cons, effects on the baby, as well as the progress of your labor. If you approach this stage of your pregnancy with your mind made up one way or the other, you are making a mistake. Keep an open mind. Get all the facts. Make sure your partner knows what might happen, too.

The pain of childbirth is caused by your contracting uterus, the surrounding muscles swelling to their maximum, and the cervix being pulled open wide. During the early stages, this pain can feel like dull aches in your groin area or lower back. When your labor is in full stride, the pains can be very uncomfortable. There's a brief period called *transition* that arrives at the end of the first stage of labor when labor pains are arriving every minute, which I would consider the most painful. You can feel overwhelmed, nauseous, horrible, cranky, willing to give up or give anything to be somewhere else and out of pain. Fortunately, this phase only lasts a short time, up to a half hour for most women. After transition when your cervix is opened fully and you start pushing, the sensations change. The hardest work I've ever done was pushing my first baby out into the world, and while it hurt, the pain seemed to have a purpose. I was working hard to meet this new little person. Some women recall the feeling of this pushing stage as more of a burning sensation than a painful one.

Anthropologist Margaret Mead wrote about the pain of her child's birth in 1939 in her book *Blackberry Winter* because she was surprised. "All night I felt as if I were getting an attack of malaria, but I did not know—one of those things one does not know— whether the sensation of having a baby might not feel like malaria. And I was fascinated to discover that far from being 'ten times worse than the worst pain you ever had' (as our childless woman doctor had told us in college) or 'worse than the worst cramps you ever had, but at least you get something out of it' (as my mother had said), the pains of childbirth were altogether different from the enveloping effects of other kinds of pain. These were pains one could follow with one's mind; they were like a fine electric needle outlining one's pelvis." Plan to write down your own impressions in a few weeks after the birth. I don't remember fine electric needles at all, but I do recall the totally amazing sensation of my child's body sliding out of my own. The physical calm that arrived with that flat stomach was absolutely delicious.

Pain relief during labor and delivery falls into two categories: analgesics or anesthetics. Analgesics relax you, make you drowsy or high, and help you rest between contractions. Never having been a catnapper before, I was shocked by how I could actually fall asleep in minuscule snatches of time during labor. With analgesics, you aren't ever completely unconscious or unaware of what your convulsing body is going through. Narcotics (meperidine or Demerol, alphprodine or Nisentil), barbiturates (Seconal, Nembutal), and tranquilizers (Valium) are considered analgesics. These pain relievers, which are available right from the beginning of labor, work by depressing your system. The bad news is that they can cross the placenta and in the worst-case scenario, they can make your new baby drowsy or unresponsive at birth. However, when analgesics are carefully administered in small doses, you don't have to worry about such side effects. A little bit of Demerol, which may take twenty minutes to start working, can help you stay more relaxed for up to three hours afterward. On Demerol, women besides me, report being able to nap even for brief moments in between contractions.

Anesthetics pack a more powerful punch. According to Howard Shapiro, M.D., a Connecticut obstetrician, anesthesia will "obliterate pain either through induction of the semiconscious (general anesthesia) or by interrupting the pathway of nerves that carries sensations of pain to the brain." There are three main types of anesthesia:

- *Balanced anesthesia*, according to Dr. Shapiro, "is a combination of drugs, each dosage sufficient to produce its own desired effects, and used to achieve a light state of general anesthesia with muscle relaxation and minimal exposure of the fetus to anesthetic agents."
- With a *general anesthesia*, you completely lose consciousness, as well as the use of your muscles and reflexes. It is not used very often nowadays. Unless your birth becomes complicated, you won't actually be offered this as an option. Speak to your doctor about it, however, because in the event

Buying a Car Seat for Your Baby

A baby car seat is required by law. In fact, you won't be able to leave the hospital if you don't have one. You have the option of buying a car seat that is strictly for infants (rear-facing only and handles babies up to twenty pounds) or one that is for both infants and toddlers (can convert to front-facing and holds an infant or toddler up to forty-five pounds). A combination infant/toddler car seat will probably do the trick. Keep in mind that some of the combination seats lack portability—an important consideration for some. Some states require seats not only for car travel but for airplane as well. In vehicles with airbags in the front passenger seat, any car seat must be placed in the back seat of the car.

of a rushed, emergency cesarean section, general anesthesia might be the doctor's first choice. Sometimes in cases of fetal distress, the rapid way that a general can knock you out is exactly what's called for. Local anesthesia can take up to a half hour to take effect. However, general anesthesia is considered a poor choice because it can be dangerous for both you and your baby. Any food left in your stomach can become lethal if you vomit and aspirate it into your lungs. Newborns arriving under the influence of a general anesthesia are likely to be drowsy and depressed, too.

- *Local*, or *regional*, *anesthesia* falls into several categories, but the one you've probably heard most is an *epidural*. A *local*, as the name indicates, will numb you partially and in a particular area.

What's an Epidural?

Injected by needle into the space between two vertebrae of your lower back, the epidural space, this type of anesthetic is administered when you are well into labor and will temporarily numb the nerves all the way from your belly button to your knees. The anesthesiologist can't offer you an epidural until your labor is in the advanced stages because the important job of effacing (i.e., opening) of your cervix could be interrupted or stopped. An epidural takes

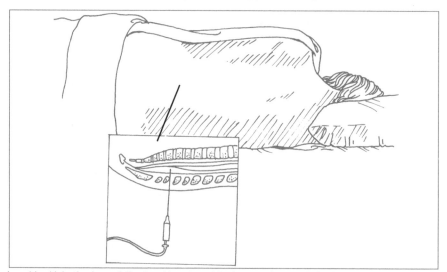

An epidural injection is carefully placed into the epidural space of your spinal column.

twenty minutes to start working and can also slow your blood pressure and make it difficult for you to know when to push.

Hooked up to an intravenous (IV) line in your arm, you will be asked to twist forward as you lie on your side to expose your spinal cord clearly for the anesthesiologist. Your lower back will be antiseptically cleaned and you may be asked to push your neck forward so your spine and its vertebrae become as clearly differentiated as possible. This can be hard to do if you are in the middle of contractions and your belly is also in the way, but the specialist wants to put the needle between your fourth and fifth lumbar vertebrae, in your lower back. The anesthesia, a small dose at first, is injected through a tiny plastic, hollow tube (catheter), which has been inserted. The anesthesia does not go directly into your spinal cord, nor will it enter the baby's bloodstream at all. As soon as the first dose starts to work and your uterus becomes a little numb, another dose is injected. You may feel a little stinging sensation down your legs, but your breathing and the involuntary muscles working those contractions won't be affected. The doctor may wrap the tube, which is sticking into your back, in something soft and then tape it to your skin so you are all set for more medication when you need it without the mess or stress of contorting your body into uncomfortable positions. If you have an epidural, your vital signs will be monitored closely to make sure that you're okay and that labor and the timing of contractions don't slow up too much.

The numbness will take several hours to wear off and may restrict your movements during the birth, but an epidural could be exactly what you need to help your baby out. You may feel faint later or have a headache. Yet, scores of new moms swear that an epidural is the only way to deliver because they feel no pain but can be wide awake to meet their child. Meanwhile others insist that you have to wait so long into labor that you might as well go the distance without this type of anesthesia.

If a Caudal is Suggested

Like an epidural, a caudal block will relieve your pain when medication enters your body through a tube inserted in your lower spine. *Caudal* actually means "tail," and the anesthesiologist will put the needle into the bony area right at the end of your spine. Caudals used to be more popular, but doctors like Shapiro explain that administering the medication is trickier because of the positioning of the needle, and a caudal can slow labor down because your abdominal and pelvic area muscles are also directly affected. "The caudal block technique requires a great deal of skill and uses a far greater quantity of anesthetic than epidurals in order to be effective," Shapiro states.

What's a Spinal?

It's easy to confuse an epidural with a spinal. Both take full advantage of your lower back, which is the point of entry for the medicine. However, a spinal is a type of anesthesia that is delivered directly into your lower spine, not into the spaces between your vertebrae as in an epidural. Used right at delivery only or during a C-section, the spinal will numb you all the way up to your rib cage and you'll be wide awake. Spinals can slow up labor pains to the point of stopping them and can make it difficult for you to push your baby out. A bad headache can also be in store for you afterward.

Other Anesthetic Blocks

A *saddle block* is a type of low spinal that numbs a more limited area of your body. The expression comes from the fact that the parts of your body numbed are exactly those that would be in contact with a saddle if you were sitting on a horse.

In a *paracervical block* the anesthetic is injected into either side of your cervix during labor to numb the area.

In a *pudendal block* the anesthetic is administered to the nerves around the vagina and pelvic floor to help control pain when the baby's head bulges into your cervix.

Other Tools & Topics to Talk About Now

Prepping Steps

When you arrive at the hospital or birthing center, there are steps the nursing staff may routinely take to get you ready for delivery. Ask your doctor what's in store. For instance, one of the

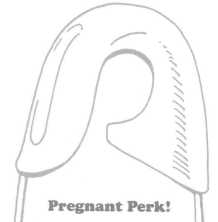

first steps in this preparation, or "prepping," routine could be having your pubic hair shaved. Years ago, hospitals actually shaved the entire stomach and abdomen area even when the presence of hair was seriously negligible. I was shocked when it happened to me and wondered why the hair around my belly button needed to be buzzed off. Some doctors explain that shaving the pubic area lessens the chance of infection and offers the delivery team a better view of the baby's arrival. Others say that the risk of infection is actually increased by the shave of such a sensitive area at such a critical time. Nowadays, most hospitals that recommend shaving, confine the procedure to a mini-prep and just shave around the vagina and the anus. The full prep does live on, however, so be sure to find out ahead of time. Speak up if you object. When your hair is growing back, the itch and stubble are pretty uncomfortable.

Another prepping step is the *enema*. Unless your labor is far advanced and the contractions are coming quite close together, the nurse may administer an enema to empty your bowels. Technically speaking, an empty bowel makes it easier for your baby to move down the birth canal, so the rationale is not completely crazy. However, having a stranger give you an enema when you are in the early stages of labor and dealing with the experience of contractions can make your first encounter with hospital policies nightmarish. Find out now what's in store and make your wishes heard loud and clear. You may even be put on a bedpan if you have been confined to your bed. An enema can also intensify your contractions. As birth and labor progress, the body seems to take care of fecal matter on its own by sending you to the toilet anyway. Some women have bouts of diarrhea early in labor, as well as episodes of vomiting. If you don't want to have an enema, speak up. If you arrive at the hospital with an empty bowel because you've been rushing back and forth to the bathroom while you time contractions, tell the nurse your bowels are already empty.

Up in Stirrups?

Some women cringe about the very notion of being stretched and strapped into delivery room table stirrups. Honestly, who would welcome such an ungraceful physical state? Other women accept this obstetrical practice as just one of those birthing issues that may not

Pregnant Perk!

Locate the Source of Your Stress

If you are feeling overwhelmed, stop and focus on the reason why. By dissecting a day's load of stress, you may be able to pinpoint a particular problem sending you over the edge of that proverbial cliff. You may even be able to deal with the stress more effectively. Too many projects on your plate at one time? All marked urgent? Before you panic, put requests on your time in order. Then, rest. Then, tackle them slowly.

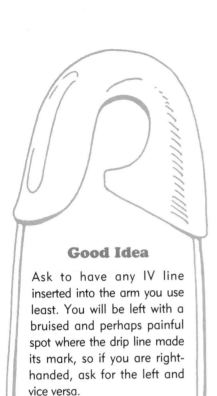

Good Idea

Ask to have any IV line inserted into the arm you use least. You will be left with a bruised and perhaps painful spot where the drip line made its mark, so if you are right-handed, ask for the left and vice versa.

be avoidable, depending upon hospital and doctor policies. Ask your practitioner where he or she fits into the debate. Stirrups are supposed to elevate your feet and legs, keeping them clear of your baby's arrival. Some practitioners still insist on having room to maneuver during those last stages of labor and delivery to make the procedure safer. However, stirrups are being used less frequently because women aren't always lying flat and confined to a delivery room table. Moreover, being prepared and knowledgeable about the most comfortable birthing positions makes you less likely to descend into an uncontrollable panic where you might kick your doctor or flail your legs at an inopportune time.

IV, Anyone?

In some hospitals you will quickly be hooked up to an intravenous line that delivers a solution of glucose and water. Analgesics and anesthetic agents can also be given through this IV line. The IV is supposed to prevent your becoming dehydrated and help maintain your blood pressure under anesthesia. In most hospitals IVs are given only if you develop complications. Your doctor may even recommend that you drink plenty of fluids before you arrive at the hospital for the birth.

You May Be Hooked Up to a Fetal Monitor

To keep close track of your baby's condition during labor, your doctor may order a fetal monitoring device. When you first climb up into bed after slipping into your laboring outfit, the doctor will want to gauge how your baby is handling the rigors of your contractions. There are two types of monitors. Both measure the fetal heart beat, recording patterns on a computer screen or old-fashioned paper-generated readout. With the external variety, known as the Doppler ultrasonic transducer, small pads placed beneath straps are positioned around your abdomen to measure your contractions and to pick up the fetal heart sounds. I can recall the sound of the regular beeps during my labor with my son, Zach. A monitor will alert you to any heart abnormalities as well as signs of oxygen deprivation or problems with the umbilical cord. Happy to know he was healthy and on his way to my arms, I was also frustrated because the machine kept me confined to bed for long hours. This type can also miss sounds.

Although more accurate, an internal fetal monitor based on the electrocardiogram, may be even more constricting because a wire is inserted up your vagina and attached to the baby's head. The most accurate internal monitors are usually reserved for high-risk pregnancies. If your practitioner recommends fetal monitoring during your labor, ask for good reasons why you need to remain strapped down.

Keep in mind that the internal is more sensitive and consistent. There is a little spiral that sits on the baby's head, which will cause a pin stick. Yet, this type of monitoring is safer. And, according to Dr. Howard Berk, "The monitor can be stopped at any time. Whether you have an acoustic or external, or an internal electronic monitor, you may want to walk around during labor." However, every fifteen minutes, you will be hooked back up to the machine and more often as you get close to delivery. "Most women, even those who are really active, don't want to do very much walking when they are having contractions every two and a half minutes, lasting a full minute. They want to be in bed then," says Berk.

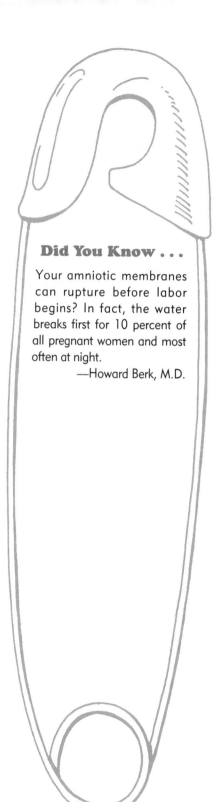

Did You Know . . .

Your amniotic membranes can rupture before labor begins? In fact, the water breaks first for 10 percent of all pregnant women and most often at night.

—Howard Berk, M.D.

Inducing Labor Could Be Proposed

Every hospital and obstetrical practice has varying policies on inducing labor or starting childbirth artificially. Sit down this month and talk about your doctor's philosophy. If you pass your due date by more than two weeks, if your blood pressure shoots up, or you develop any other condition that puts your baby at risk, induction may be a decision you'll have to make. Make sure there is a good reason for being induced.

Nine Months and Still Counting?

Generally speaking, your pregnancy may be considered past due, prolonged, or postdated when labor fails to arrive after forty-two weeks. However, not all pregnancies are correctly dated so the practitioner will perform various reassessments, including an ultrasound and fetal monitoring, to make sure you aren't being considered for labor induction too soon. If you are only thirty some weeks pregnant and your cervix isn't quite ready for delivery, then an induced labor is a bad idea. On the other hand, the consequences of letting the baby remain in the womb past forty-two weeks can be dangerous. Wastes begin to accumulate in the amniotic fluid, including the baby's green fecal matter called meconium. The umbilical cord can become compressed and obstruct oxygen to the baby. Postterm babies can have kidney problems and a higher risk of pneumonia. Some can continue to grow making vaginal delivery long and complicated because of the infant's size. However, as they grow in the womb longer, postterm babies actually lose fat and appear leaner at birth in spite of weights of ten pounds or more.

If you must be induced, you'll have a preassigned arrival time at the hospital and one of several steps may be taken:

- *Amniotomy* is the process by which the doctor will break the *amniotic sac*, the bag of fluid that has surrounded and cushioned the baby for months. Ordinarily, this bag won't break until you are well into labor. When you are induced, the doctor inserts an instrument up into your vagina and through your cervix to make a small hole in the membrane. Usually painless, the rupturing allows the water to flood out and labor pains start thereafter. According to the American College of Obstetricians and Gynecologists (ACOG), most women go into labor within twelve hours. An amniotomy is a good idea because it allows for internal monitoring and gives a view into the baby's environment and responses. The presence of meconium, which may indicate fetal distress, can be seen, according to Dr. Berk.
- *Stripping the membranes?* Your doctor may also attempt to force your body into labor using a technique known as *stripping*. This can be done in the office. Inserting a finger into the cervix, she or he will try to separate the amniotic membrane from where it is attached to the lower uterine wall.
- *Synthetic hormones* can also jumpstart labor. Hooked to an IV line in the hospital, you will be given oxytocin or pitocin. It won't take long after these agents are present in your blood stream for your uterus to swing into action and send your baby on its way. These hormones mimic normal labor.

Taking Matters into Your Own Hands

Late in delivery when, or if, labor has stalled, there are two other less dramatic and rather simplistic ways to help your uterus:

- *Get out of bed and move*. Don't remain flat on your back in a supine position if your labor has stalled. Talk with your nurse, and if she thinks it's reasonable, walk around, squat, lean upright against a wall, get into a chair, or kneel and lean forward on your hands. Even if you feel miserable moving out of bed, an upright stature can help speed labor and increase the intensity of the contractions that are forcing your baby out.

  Or, have someone prop you up. By remaining flat on your back, you may even experience a drop in blood pressure that isn't going to help you or your baby. If you must lie down, turn to your left side. The old-fashioned, standard position for delivering a baby in a hospital, known technically as the *lithotomy position*, is definitely not the best, especially if you want to keep your baby moving out. Even if you feel downright sick, have someone help you up so the force of gravity can work with your own efforts to push. The baby's head will be able to press on your cervix and stimulate your own hormones to produce more oxytocin, which causes the contractions, naturally.

- *Stimulate your nipples*. When the nipples and areolas of your breasts are stimulated using the palm of the hand, you can create a hormonal chain of reactions that produces oxytocin in your body naturally. Once considered an old-wives' tale and mentioned in nineteenth-century obstetric texts, some modern moms and doctors have investigated the process and found that it can work. You can use not only your hands, but also hot towels or a breast pump. The hormonal release can strengthen contractions that may have slowed down. The same biological process is at work when you breastfeed and your baby sucks on your nipples to release the hormone that lets your milk flow freely. Although there are reports of women trying nipple stimulation during this last ninth month on their own to hurry matters along, don't go this route without discussing the idea with your practitioner.

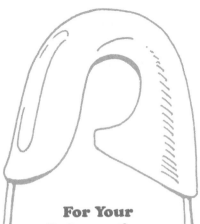

Forceps were first called "mains de fer," which translates from French into "hands of iron." According to author Rebecca Rowe Parfitt, in *The Birth Primer*, they have been around since 1588, when two English brothers, the Chamberlens, invented them. Secretive, melodramatic characters, the Chamberlens were so afraid someone would steal their invention that they would arrive on the scene of a difficult birth with their special tool hidden in a chest. After charging an exorbitant fee and ordering everyone else from the scene of the birth, they would blindfold the laboring woman and hastily pull her baby out. Midwives, who hated the very idea of this metal manipulation, protested and insisted that "hands of flesh" were far more appropriate.

Can Forceps Help Guide Your Baby Out?

If your labor slows up, if your baby shows signs of distress, if you can't push a moment longer near the very end of your delivery experience, and if your cervix is fully open with your baby's head naturally engaged, the doctor may choose to use forceps. Standard practice is to let you push for two hours. If there is no progress and your baby isn't making progress in the descent down and out of the birth canal, then you may need some assistance. These metal instruments can speed such a stalled delivery along by allowing the doctor to reach up into your birth canal and gently tug the baby out. The tool, which is not used routinely as it once was, looks a little like tongs with two big open-scooped spoons attached to one handle. The scoops of each spoon gently attach to the sides of your baby's head so the doctor can pull the baby through the birth canal while you keep on pushing. If it looks as if you require a forceps delivery, the doctor will administer local anesthesia to your pelvic floor area. However, an epidural or a spinal are usually better, according to Dr. Berk.

Although forceps gained a nasty reputation over the years, the mention of this instrument should not send shivers up your spine. Forceps can actually protect a baby's head from pressure and damage during a difficult delivery. When a baby is arriving prematurely, when the head is simply too large for you to deliver (known as *cephalopelvic disproportion* or CPD), or there are other complications, the skilled use of forceps can hasten the birth process.

Forceps are also used to reposition a baby who is intent on arriving in a poor position. The doctor may be able to shift the baby, and forceps can also help protect a baby from your powerful pushing right up against the perineum. You may hear the expressions a *high, mid, or low forceps* delivery and these simply indicate whether the doctor inserts the instrument high into the birth canal or lower. When forceps are used at all, the low position is more likely than any other. Sometimes forceps are simply used to lift the baby up and out right there at your perineum, which is called *perineal use.* Babies delivered via forceps do wear signs of these instruments as bruises or red marks on either side of their heads for a few days and there is a very remote risk of brain injury. Yet, modern-day use of forceps can be quite safe. In the hands of a trained obstetrician, they are nothing to fear.

Vacuum Extraction as an Option at Delivery Time

First used in Sweden, the vacuum extractor is a pump that can be placed on the baby's head near the very end of your labor to help pull a stubborn baby into the light of day. If your baby is large, if your labor has slowed up, if you are unable to push your baby out, and if the fit inside the birth canal is so tight that the doctor worries that using forceps might tear up tissue, the vacuum extraction may be an option. You will need an episiotomy and local anesthesia, of course. Ask your obstetrician about his use of a vacuum extractor because skill will be important. Suctioned onto the baby's head, the cup is attached to a chain that the doctor pulls on while you keep on pushing. The cup will simply fall off the baby's head if too much pressure builds up. However, babies who arrive via vacuum extraction can have a bruised, swollen look to the top of their heads. There's no risk of brain damage, though.

Exactly What Is an Episiotomy?

When the skin of your vaginal opening won't stretch far enough, to make it easier for your baby's head to arrive outside without tearing the edges, the doctor may decide to make a small cut. Called an *episiotomy*, this little snip is made into your perineum, the area between your vagina and your anus. Most episiotomies are medial and not to the right or the left. Median is the mid-line. Right media-lateral will go to the right. Left media-lateral will go to the left. However, those are used most often with only very difficult deliveries or with someone who has a short perineal area.

Bring up the issue of episiotomies now. Ask your doctor what his or her philosophy is on the practice. An episiotomy can be necessary if your baby is being delivered breech, if he or she is premature, distressed, or the head is large. When forceps are being used or any other special assistance, this kind of cut may also be called for.

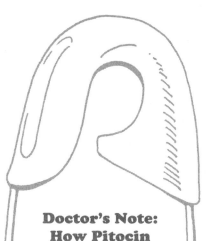

Doctor's Note: How Pitocin Works

Prostaglandins are naturally occurring substances that cause strong contractions of the smooth muscles in your body and dilatation of certain vascular beds. You can find prostaglandins in menstrual blood. Most experts believe that pitocin causes the release of prostaglandins and when it reaches a certain level, it takes over and causes the contractions. As Dr. Berk explains, "I can even turn off the pitocin and labor contractions will continue." The amount of pitocin that you need is probably that which causes the release of prostaglandins.

If you haven't had any local anesthesia up to this point, it will be administered to your pelvic floor at the height of a contraction, and just before the baby's head is delivered. Your skin is so stretched and numb near delivery that you may not feel anything at all. A few stitches after the birth will close the cut. Don't hesitate to ask for more anesthesia at this point if you feel pain because the repair work can hurt more after the birth than it did during the delivery. Although small, the stitches have to sew together bands of muscle as well as several layers of skin. Healing can be a real pain—literally in the butt. For about two weeks, you'll be sore, need to take warm baths, and perhaps even rely on heat lamp treatments. Infections from episiotomy cuts can also develop. Some studies claim that healing from a small tear is less painful than an episiotomy. However, controversy about episiotomies is ongoing. If you are concerned, ask your practitioner. To avoid an episiotomy, you may also want to learn and practice relaxation exercises for your pelvic floor to help the skin stretch naturally when under pressure. Staying up on your feet during labor and delivery can help make the need for an episiotomy less likely.

To avoid the need for an episiotomy, some practitioners may also attempt to massage the perineum and apply finger pressure just at the point when the baby's head has descended. You may have even heard this technique referred to as "ironing out the perineum," but the results are mixed. In fact, some women find the massage an irritating intrusion.

"As an obstetrician, my feeling about episiotomies is that a properly placed episiotomy is easier to repair than a large laceration and a properly placed episiotomy can replace future vaginal plastic surgery," says Dr. Berk.

In a Do-It-Yourself, Emergency Birth

My neighbor had four children, and with each birth her labor and delivery became shorter and shorter. The last time, she claims that the baby nearly popped out when she knelt down on the bathroom floor alongside the tub while giving her three preschoolers their

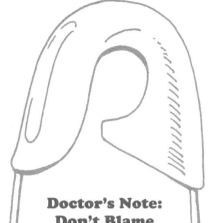

nightly bath. Stories of babies being born in taxi-cabs, on airplanes, in the back seat of cars, delivered by shaky husbands, cabbies, policemen, and complete strangers are legendary, but probably not nearly as common as you might suspect. Nevertheless, if you find yourself out of time near the pushing stage of labor, these emergency tips may come in handy for the people around you. As the expectant mom in the middle of this crisis, you may not be in any condition to read. Thus, the advice is for your next-of-kin or soon-to-be close friend:

- You don't have to be a professionally trained obstetrician or midwife to help a baby be born. Relax. Stay calm. Call 911 if you have access to a phone so back-up medical care will be on the way. Don't wait to dial. As soon as you suspect that you will be unable to reach a hospital or birthing center in time for the delivery, call.
- Have the mother lie back or stretch out on a bed, car seat, table, or desktop with her knees up, her underpants off, and her back supported in some way. Lying down may actually slow down the delivery. If possible, cover the surface beneath her hips and under her thighs with clean towels, plastic, or paper.
- Have the mother keep her knees up and spread apart, and check to see if the baby's head is visible.
- Keep a soft, reassuring tone of voice. Don't stop talking to the mother, who may be very frightened. Reach for a confident banter. Say: "You can do it. We can do it. Don't worry. Help is on the way. Everything is under control. There's nothing we can't do together here."
- Ask the mom to pant as you gather a few essentials. Can you find any clean cloth to wrap the baby (clean sheets? a blanket? a shirt? your coat?)? Shoelaces or string for tying the umbilical cord? Scissors for cutting the cord? A syringe to suck mucus from the newborn's air passages? The panting will help the laboring woman stop pushing and slow up the baby's arrival. Any makeshift instruments should really be sterilized in boiling water if you are at home and

Doctor's Note: Don't Blame Pitocin

My basic belief is that if labor is indicated, pitocin is indicated. Take the example of a woman who has been "piddling" along in labor, having very delightful contractions every ten minutes, I'll say, "Look, you've been four centimeters dilated for three hours. I have to do something for you." Then, if I give her pitocin, the pitocin is blamed for producing what is actually a normal labor. That's all that pitocin does.

—Howard Berk, M.D.

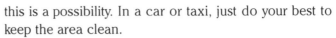

this is a possibility. In a car or taxi, just do your best to keep the area clean.

- Whoever is going to catch, or actually deliver, the baby should wash his or her hands. Meanwhile, this person should stand or crouch to one side of the mom and allow the baby to arrive as naturally as possible. No pulling or tugging are needed.

- As the head emerges, the person delivering should put his or her hand just beneath the baby's head, gently cradling as the little body turns and shoulders begin to appear.

- Check to see if the umbilical cord is wrapped around the neck. If it is, unloop or loosen it slightly. If possible, tug it very lightly up or off. If the cord is just loosely wrapped, you may not need to be concerned for the moment. Don't yank it because of the risk of hemorrhage. Don't panic. Keep talking.

- You will want to help the baby release any mucus, blood, or fluids from the nose and respiratory tract. If you found a little ear bulb syringe, squeeze the bulb, place it gently in the baby's nose, release, and pull the contents out. With no syringe, try stroking the little nose in a downward motion with the tips of your fingers. The idea is to loosen and rid the contents stuck in the nostrils. Holding the head down also helps fluids drain.

- As the mother is still pushing and you are gently cupping the baby's head down and out of her body, you'll see first one shoulder and then the other emerge. The rest of the body should slip out easily. Lift the head and body up. You don't need to yank or slap the baby's bottom. Just make sure that the nose and mouth are clear so those first breaths of life are not being hindered in any way. As soon as the baby takes in oxygen from the air and gives off carbon dioxide, the route of the blood in the umbilical cord changes direction. The incredible importance of the placenta, still inside the mother, starts to diminish.

- Very gently, without pulling, wrap the baby in something warm and clean. Put him or her right up next to the mother's breast if the cord is long enough. If it won't stretch that far, just up on her abdomen or even on her thigh will be fine for a few minutes.

- The cord should be pulsing with the exchange of blood and oxygen. Don't try to tie it or cut it for the time being. At this point, you may even want to just sit tight until help arrives.

- Keep the mother and her baby as warm as possible. The drop in temperature for the newborn has been dramatic because inside the womb it was warm and wet. Let the mom attempt to breastfeed because the stimulation to her nipple will speed up the third stage of labor, the delivery of the placenta.

- Within the next half hour, the placenta will be expelled. You can help the mother by massaging her stomach near the top of the uterus to keep her contractions coming. This also helps stop the bleeding. Don't pull the cord in any attempt to loosen the placenta. If it arrives without your intervention, wrap it in something and hold it higher than the baby.

- If no help arrives and the cord has definitely stopped throbbing, you can tie a shoelace or piece of string or cloth tightly around it, halfway between the mother or her placenta and the baby. Tie a second piece two to three inches away from your first. Cutting the cord between the two ties should be safe.

- Babies are individuals right at birth. Some cry loudly. Some urinate. Some have eyes wide open in wonder. Others arrive hungry or anxious for a mother's breast. Some yawn, stretch, hiccup, and appear to wonder what in the world has happened to them.

I Was Wondering . . .

I keep hearing about Apgar Scores. Is this a test my baby will have to take so soon in life?

Yes, it's a test given twice within the first few moments of your baby's life to assess physical condition and alert the doctors to possible emergencies. When Dr. Virginia Apgar was working as a

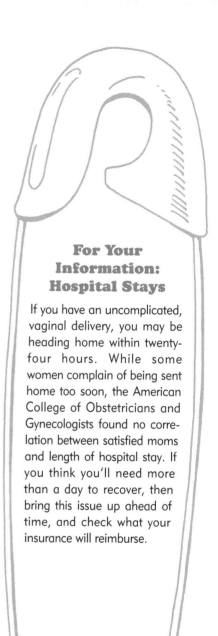

For Your Information: Hospital Stays

If you have an uncomplicated, vaginal delivery, you may be heading home within twenty-four hours. While some women complain of being sent home too soon, the American College of Obstetricians and Gynecologists found no correlation between satisfied moms and length of hospital stay. If you think you'll need more than a day to recover, then bring this issue up ahead of time, and check what your insurance will reimburse.

professor of anesthesiology at New York's Columbia-Presbyterian Hospital in the early 1950s, she took part in the births of thousands of babies. Obstetricians would ask her to assess the newborn's condition; and to make the process more methodical and efficient, she came up with a test based on the letters in her last name. *A* for *a*ppearance or skin color; *P* for *p*ulse; *G* for *g*rimace or reflexes; *A* for *a*ctivity; and *R* for *r*espiration. First published formally in 1953, her very personal "newborn scoring system" is so famous that it even appears in dictionaries now as her name in lower case. Just one minute after birth, the birth attendant will assign a score of 0 to 2 for each category. Then, a second assessment is made five minutes later. Most babies' score for all five categories is between 7 and 10, and many do better on the second test, which is a bit more accurate as a predictor of health. The shock of birth can take a few seconds to recover from, after all. To give you an idea of the range of ranking within each category, a blue or pale appearance would rate a 0, while a completely pink baby would get a 2. An infant with a pulse rate less than 100 beats per minute would be considered slow and get a 1, while another with a heart rate above 100 beats per minute would earn a 2. If your baby was crying loudly, a score of 2 would be registered for respiration. Scoring is rather subjective, however, and the Apgar score is only one method of evaluating a newborn baby. Some doctors have a longer checklist to rate the babies they deliver. Ask your obstetrician if he relies on Apgar alone or uses any other measures.

What's a delivery room really like?

Old-fashioned delivery rooms used to be pretty inhospitable places: cold metal, reverberating sounds, bright lights, hard surgical tables that were very unforgiving for women about to give birth. Decor has definitely changed as hospitals compete for pregnant couples' business, but still, if it's possible to stay right in the room where you've been spending labor, do so. Although many delivery rooms are no longer as sterile and uncomfortable, you should take an advance look because they still vary tremendously from hospital to hospital. When you go for the tour, make sure you don't skip the delivery room. What's probably far more troubling than the decor of the delivery room is the time that your transfer takes place: right at the end, when you don't feel like taking your mind off the birth process at hand. You may be wheeled away for this transfer when your cervix is either fully dilated to ten centimeters or at seven to eight centimeters. First-time moms stay in the labor room longer because pushing ordinarily takes longer. No matter when you make the switch, it will feel as if you are at the very end of labor and you may be at your worst phase physically. Ask the doctor how many quick moves you will have to make to get to the delivery room. The hospital may have a transporting table that doubles as a delivery table, eliminating the need to switch from labor bed to moving vehicle and then to operating room or delivery room table. The lights are usually bright in a delivery room, and the waist-high table is equipped with leg stirrups so your legs can be raised high up in the air, exposing your vagina area fully for the doctor. If you don't want to climb into stirrups, object now while you still have all your wits about you and hospital personnel don't dismiss your wishes. On the table, you may be lying on your back or positioned into a half-sit. Take pillows with you for back support. Ask your mate or the nurse to hold your back up. In the old days, wrists were also strapped down. Don't let anyone strap your wrists. Hospitals have become hip to what expectant moms really need now and some have taken the medicalese decor out of the rooms. However, in an emergency, decorative extras are not going to make you feel as confident as having all the modern medical equipment to keep you and your baby safe.

I understand that I won't be able to eat or drink anything during labor. This seems just crazy. Why is it standard practice to starve expectant moms?

Laboring women are not supposed to eat or drink during labor because digestion itself shuts down when you are giving birth. Anything you eat or drink will just sit there in your gastrointestinal

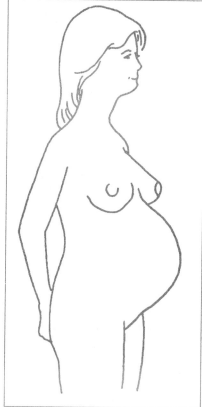

By the final week of pregnancy, your skin will feel stretched and taut across your abdomen, as the baby is at maximum size.

tract causing digestive problems, crowding the uterus, which is hard at work, or making you feel sick either with nausea or diarrhea. Another reason why food and liquids are off limits is because in the event of an emergency and the need to administer general anesthesia, whatever remains in your stomach could make you vomit and you could choke or inhale the vomitus. You can see why this standard practice is not really so crazy. Having said that, I must admit that laboring for hour after hour takes a lot of energy and sometimes women in labor lose strength, not just because of the physical effort, but also because they need nourishment to keep going. In European hospitals, women are allowed light snacks, juices, and broths. Ask your practitioner how she or he feels about light snacks or juices during early labor. Some recommend only ice chips for laboring women and others prohibit everything but fluids via an IV line.

I can't decide whether to choose "rooming-in" and have my baby by my side. I may be so exhausted that I'll need to sleep without worrying about the baby. What's the best option?

There is no right or wrong option here. First check with the hospital to see what kind of policies they have regarding recovery and newborn care. "Rooming-in," or keeping the baby by your side in your hospital room twenty-four hours a day, is a nice option if you think you'll want as much quiet time as possible with your new baby while you are still under the watchful eyes of trained baby nurses. Rest assured that no matter what you decide, you won't be completely on your own while you are still in the hospital. If you need sleep, you can always ask the staff to take the baby for a few hours. You may be able to keep the baby with you during the day and opt for the ease of night time nursery care. Unless you have emergency surgery, you won't really be in the hospital for very long after all. Perhaps a good night's sleep will be something that your body desperately requires after the work of labor.

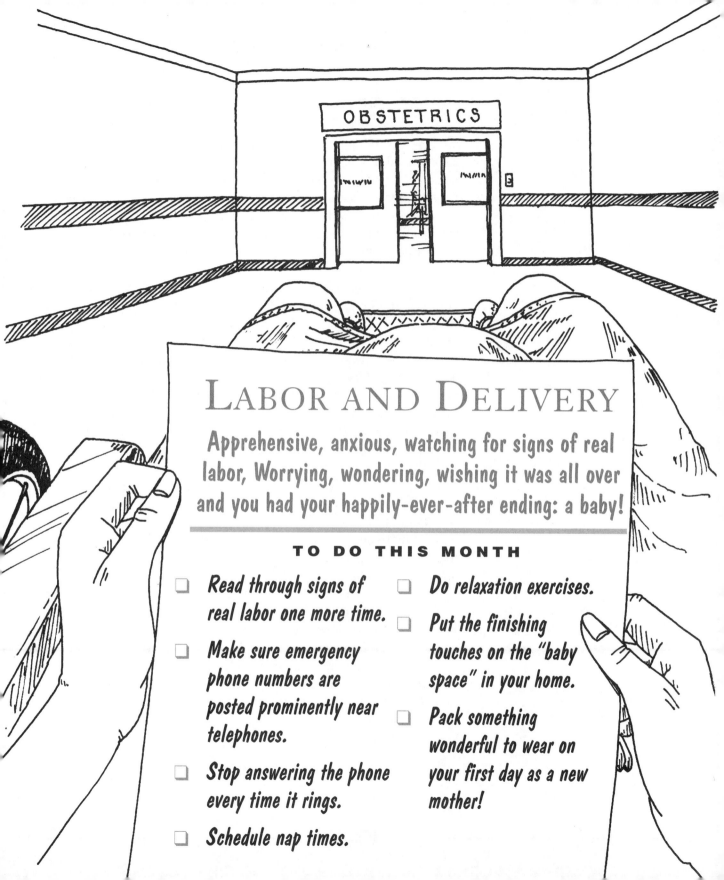

LABOR AND DELIVERY

Apprehensive, anxious, watching for signs of real labor, Worrying, wondering, wishing it was all over and you had your happily-ever-after ending: a baby!

TO DO THIS MONTH

- ☐ Read through signs of real labor one more time.

- ☐ Make sure emergency phone numbers are posted prominently near telephones.

- ☐ Stop answering the phone every time it rings.

- ☐ Schedule nap times.

- ☐ Do relaxation exercises.

- ☐ Put the finishing touches on the "baby space" in your home.

- ☐ Pack something wonderful to wear on your first day as a new mother!

My first "giving-birth" day arrived by surprise two weeks earlier than estimated by my obstetrician. I was still working full time and looking forward to my pre-baby vacation. All my plans for resting and getting organized evaporated on a Friday afternoon while I was at my desk in New York City. A strange trickling sensation and wet underpants had plagued me all morning, but it was a warm day in May and I chalked off the discharge to excess mucus as usual. My mission to bring order to my office before I departed for maternity leave was finally brought to a cold stop when the leak got larger. The wetness became impossible to shrug off. Yet, there was no flood. How could it be amniotic fluid? I remember wondering. Wasn't that supposed to gush out much later when I was into labor at full swing. Wrong! What I soon learned in my obstetrician's office was that every woman's childbirth experience can be slightly different. A high leak in the amniotic fluid sac—something I had never anticipated—was sending a clear signal that my baby was on his way out into the world. Contractions didn't even begin until later that evening after my husband Bob and I decided to go to the movies to take our minds off the impending event. Zach was born the next afternoon.

No matter how happy you may be to have these long months of waiting over, those first signs of real labor can be unsettling. Oh, you may want to say: Do I really have to do this? Can't I put it off until another more convenient time? When I told the nurse at the hospital that I had changed my mind about giving birth after all, she laughed and said, "This baby will be here shortly."

If this is your first baby, you may wonder, as I did, if you'll be able to recognize true labor at all. You may also be lulled into thinking that your delivery date is a point in time toward which you will be able to keep on going. Two weeks to go? All the time in the world to get organized? Aren't most first babies late? Hardly! I assumed that I would be late, not two weeks early! Don't wait until the last minute to start packing or planning for your baby's life at home.

Let's Get Physical
Is It the Real Thing? Signs of Labor

- Your baby drops way down low into your pelvis. This may happen weeks, days, or just hours before your body shifts into labor, but the result of *lightening*—that's what it's called— is more breathing space for you. Take a deep breath. Relax. The baby's head is positioned in your pelvis and knocking at the door to the outside world, making it difficult for you to walk or put your thighs together . . . a strange sensation, for sure, but one that won't last long.

- A blob of thick, blood-stained mucus lands on your under-pants. While you were pregnant, a thick plug of mucus accumulated at the neck of your cervix. As the cervix starts to open, the plug is eliminated, giving you one of the clearest signs that labor is on its way even if you haven't had any powerful contractions yet. The plug can actually be pink, clear, or just slightly bloody, but most experts call this sign the *bloody show*. It can happen several days before labor begins, at the very onset, or during the first stage of child-birth when your contractions are still fairly far apart.

- You may have diarrhea. Not all women end up with the rum-bling, growling, racing-to-the-bathroom diarrhea near the end of their pregnancies; but if you do, you'll know that a physio-logical chain reaction has begun. Your body seems to be making space and getting ready for childbirth. Several factors can cause diarrhea: hormones, the pressure of your baby's body on your cervix, and the push for space in your pelvis all affect your digestive system.

- Your water breaks into a trickle or a real gush of amniotic fluid. The rupture of your membranes, the thin, fluid-filled sac that has protected your unborn baby for so many months, can happen slowly, dramatically fast, or not until the baby is nearly born. The pressure of your growing baby and the stretched, contracting uterus can cause a leak in the bag. Take note of the color of this warm, salty fluid. Most of the time, it's clear, but the color can be stained with signs of

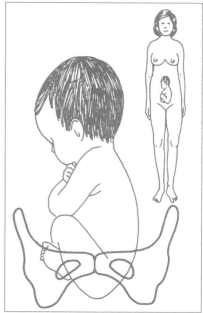

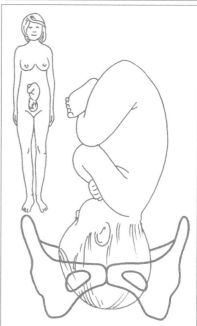

Top: The most common breech postion.

Bottom: The most common and the most desireable correct position.

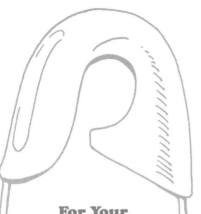

For Your Information

Uterine contractions are involuntary, of course. You don't have control over when they begin or end. Like a muscle spasm in your calf after too much exercise or hiccups, the muscle fibers contract, squeeze, actually shorten, and clamp down on the surrounding tissues or blood vessels. You've got three sets of muscles in your uterus, running up, down, and around. During labor, the longitudinal muscles pull, tighten, and push down on the baby. A middle muscle layer contracts to squeeze the blood in and out of the lining of the uterus. The third set of muscles is located down around your cervix and has kept it closed tightly up until now.

meconium and appear greenish or brown. *Meconium* is the technical name for the contents of your unborn baby's bowels and intestinal tract, so the color indicates that the baby had a bowel movement while in uterus. Sometimes it may indicate fetal distress. Don't worry. Just tell your doctor or midwife. Sometimes this sac doesn't break at all until just before birth.

- Contractions arrive in a regular, predictable pattern. Your uterus is a muscle that tightens, relaxes, and reacts to the stress of having been stretched to the outer limits with the unborn baby's growth. Your hormones, as you may have noticed all too personally, shift into high gear when you are pregnant. Progesterone seems to stabilize your uterus and estrogen has the opposite effect. From the seventh month on, some experts believe that estrogen has the upper hand in the physiological playing field of your body. As estrogen levels increase, you have more and more contractions. You may even be familiar with the Braxton-Hicks variety. When you start to have regular contractions—a tightening and then a release—anywhere from twenty to forty-five minutes apart, you know you've entered the first phase of labor. You may also have low back pain or sharp pains down your thighs.

First Stage
Early in Labor

Lots of things are happening to your body during this first stage of labor. Doctors break this stage into three parts: early, active, and transition.

- First-time moms should probably count on at least twelve to fourteen hours. If this is your second or third birth, you may luck out and spend only six to seven hours working through these tough, but bearable, contractions. You don't need to rush to the hospital or birthing center after your first contraction.
- Your cervix, which has been tightly closed during pregnancy, effaces, flattens, or thins out to become "ripe" for birth.

Effacement for a first baby can actually take place without your even sensing a change and may be complete before the cervix starts to open or dilate. Moreover, if you are already a mother, then effacement doesn't have to be 100 percent complete before your cervix starts to cooperate in the process of dilation:

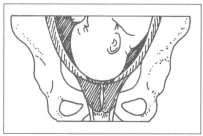

The tough cervix gradually softens to let the baby's head through.

- Effacement, the thinning-out of the cervix opening, is often described in terms of percentages and when you hear someone say that you are 100 percent effaced, you know that your cervix is ready to become part of the birth canal.
- Dilation is always measured in centimeters up to ten, which is the largest dimension of the head of most babies. If you hear the doctor or midwife describe you as almost fully dilated, you will know that your cervix is gradually stretching to that ten-centimeter opening. Midwives will use their fingers—two cm per finger—to gauge dilation, so you may hear the expression, "She's two fingers dilated." Some women actually begin to dilate during the last two to three weeks of pregnancy, making labor a lot shorter in those last bouts toward childbirth.

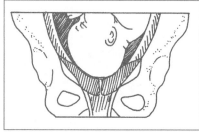

Effacement begins as the length of the cervix shortens.

- In early, or what may be called "inactive" labor, your cervix should dilate to about four or five centimeters. Contractions arrive every fifteen to twenty minutes and last sixty to ninety seconds.

What to Do

- Call your doctor or midwife. Until your contractions start arriving every five minutes or they are very painful, you may not need to go to the hospital. However, the hospital or birthing center will want to be alerted to your upcoming "birth-day" and that you may soon be on your way. Paperwork and red-tape may be able to be settled before you arrive. You will certainly not feel like talking or straightening out any last-minute insurance details. Your mind must stay focused on riding the waves of your contractions. You'll want to be paying attention to your body, not hospital administration procedures.

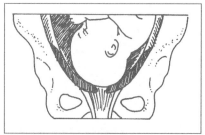

Dialation begins as the opening of the cervix increases.

- Stay up and stay home if you can. Make sure that your mate, labor coach, or best friend is nearby and ready to help when and if the going gets rough. Deep relaxed breathing will help keep you calm and open the muscles around your cervix. You want the full pressure of your baby's little body pressing down on your cervix, so don't lie back. You provide a better oxygen supply to your baby, who is working hard to emerge, because blood flow slows when you are on your back. The return of freshly oxygenated blood to your uterus must travel through your vena cava. When you are flat on your back, this vein is compressed by the weight of the uterus.

- Try to rest in between contractions, especially if labor has begun in the middle of the night. No matter how hyped up you may be about the birth, force yourself to rest now. Later, you will be happy I told you so. Eat something. You need food for energy to complete all the work ahead of you. Don't eat a humongous meal, however. That will only make you sick. A light snack, juices, or clear soup may give you a little boost. What you don't want to do is overload your digestive system with a big meal now. It will either come up or come out sooner or later.

- Don't take any medication for the pain now. You may want or be scheduled for pain relief once you arrive at the hospital or birthing center, but popping anything on your own is not recommended. Put a hot water bottle on your lower back, your abdomen, or your vagina to relieve some of the distress.

How to Handle the Discomfort . . . Sort of

- Put a pillow on the floor directly up against a chair, table, or surface that is chest-high for you when kneeling. Put another pillow on the chair, table, or flat surface. Now, kneel down with your knees slightly parted, lean forward, cross your arms, and rest your head on the flat surface.

- Take an armless chair and put a pillow on the seat. Put a second bed pillow up against the back of the chair. Sit facing the back of the chair so that your legs are spread to either side of the chair seat. Cross your arms and rest your head on the back pillow. Keep breathing deeply.

- Put a pile of pillows—more than two or three—on your bed or a firm but soft surface. Kneel down with your knees apart and lean forward onto the pile. Cross your arms and rest your head. Close your eyes. This kind of position takes the baby's weight off your back. Rock your pelvis up and then down in cat like stretches.

- On this same flat, but firm, surface, eliminate the pillow pile and kneel up firmly on all fours during a contraction. If your bed mattress is too soft, look for an exercise mat or quilt. Try not to arch your back. Keep your spine straight. When the contraction passes, lean forward in what yoga instructors refer to as the child's pose.

- Stand up during a contraction and lean up against someone you love. Rest your arms on his or her arms and keep your feet apart. Have your partner give you a back massage in this position.

- If back labor is making you miserable, have someone give you a lower back massage using the heel of the hand and dusting powder so the movements are freer and more fluid. Back labor can be caused by a baby arriving with his or her face toward your abdomen. When this happens, the baby's head presses firmly on your spine, giving you a royal back-ache during contractions when the pressure is on.

- Don't think past the very contraction you are living through. You are riding waves of discomfort, but they will pass. Tell people around you to stay calm and to let you concentrate.

- Fix your eyes on something beautiful or relaxing during contractions.

- Let out your discomfort with your voice. Don't be afraid to growl, moan, cry out, or sing. There's no need to be embarrassed. Your boisterous, natural release can help lessen the pain. Even sighing and yawning will give you extra air when your body needs the oxygen to keep on laboring. So open your mouth. Let it all out.

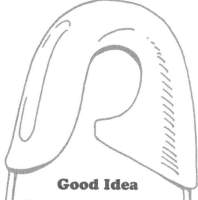

Good Idea

Time your contractions. Use a clock or watch with a second hand so you can jot down the exact time one begins and ends. Do so for at least an hour. Are the contractions at least forty seconds long? Also, real labor contractions don't stop if you move around and may start around near the bottom of your spine. Can you follow this gripping sensation as it moves around to the front and clasps hold of your abdomen? Real contractions also increase steadily in strength, growing closer together as well. There will be a rhythm to your contractions in this first stage. Even if you aren't hooked up to a monitor that can actually record the slow, wavelike pattern of this dramatic rhythmical activity, you will sense the slow buildup to a peak of intensity about halfway through. Then, the contraction declines.

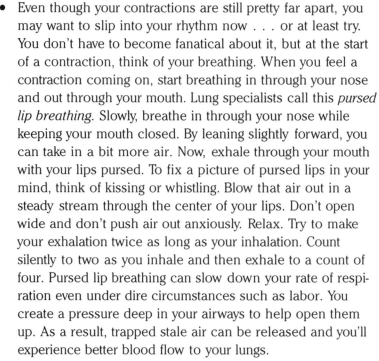

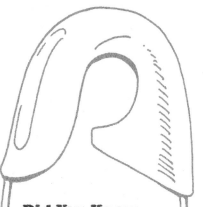

Did You Know . . .

Your uterus is a muscle that reacts to the hormones in your body. Near the end of pregnancy, the level of estrogen rises, heralding and influencing the arrival of labor contractions.

Midwives use their fingers—two centimeters per finger—to describe how labor is progressing.

A full bladder or bowel can inhibit the baby's progress down the birth canal.

Pushing your baby out of your vagina has been likened to pushing a grand piano across a large warehouse floor all by yourself.

- Even though your contractions are still pretty far apart, you may want to slip into your rhythm now . . . or at least try. You don't have to become fanatical about it, but at the start of a contraction, think of your breathing. When you feel a contraction coming on, start breathing in through your nose and out through your mouth. Lung specialists call this *pursed lip breathing*. Slowly, breathe in through your nose while keeping your mouth closed. By leaning slightly forward, you can take in a bit more air. Now, exhale through your mouth with your lips pursed. To fix a picture of pursed lips in your mind, think of kissing or whistling. Blow that air out in a steady stream through the center of your lips. Don't open wide and don't push air out anxiously. Relax. Try to make your exhalation twice as long as your inhalation. Count silently to two as you inhale and then exhale to a count of four. Pursed lip breathing can slow down your rate of respiration even under dire circumstances such as labor. You create a pressure deep in your airways to help open them up. As a result, trapped stale air can be released and you'll experience better blood flow to your lungs.

- At the peak of a contraction, go for shallow little breaths in and out of your mouth. Reserve these quick puffs in and out for the peak only because doing this for a long time can make you lightheaded or dizzy.

- Go to the bathroom often. A full bladder or bowel inhibits the baby's movement down the birth canal, so sit down on the toilet regularly even when you don't feel like you have to go. You may surprise yourself.

Relaxation Tips

Relaxation exercises are wonderful for expectant moms. If you've ever taken a yoga class, you already know just how certain simple movements and mantras can send relief to wildly stressed muscles. Most prepared childbirth classes teach relaxation tricks too. By practicing these exercises often, you will be able to respond immediately to the stress of labor. What you want your body to be able to do is to shift into relaxation mode at the first sign of stress almost without thinking. You will give your muscles an automatic memory of what to do when lightning strikes if you practice enough.

Are you comfortable? Loosen any tight clothing. Pile up pillows on a soft rug or mat. Put on soft music. Light an aromatic candle. Ignore the telephone. Because you are pregnant, you'll want to keep your chest and head higher than your lower torso so the pillows will act as your prop against your back even as you lie down. Close your eyes. Lean into the soft pillows. Put your arms and hands at your side with the palms comfortably open and up. Start with your toes. Tighten, curl them, and then relax. Bend your feet, forcing your toes to reach up tightly. Then let go. As you'll notice, this whole series of relaxation exercises is a series of tightening muscles and then relaxing the same groups. Moving up your leg, tense your calves and then relax. Go slow. Tighten your thighs and then let go. Squeeze your backside muscles. Let go. Relax. Try to pull in your stomach muscles. Then let go. Move to your hands. Make fists, squeezing, squeezing your fingers into your palms. Then, open up. Let your hands flop open. Arch your back. Tighten the muscles. Then let go. Squeeze and pull your shoulders up alongside your neck. Tighten and relax. Think about your face. Squint. Open and close your eyes. Clench your teeth together. Then let go. Move your head gently from side to side, back and forth. Let your head fall to the pillow on one side. Hold it there. Gradually move to the other side. Hold it. Then move your face forward again, keeping your eyes closed. Empty your mind of thoughts of labor and delivery. Be calm. Think of the most peaceful vacation you've ever had. Or, better yet, what's your happiest memory? Bring it back and put it in your mind's eye.

Active Labor

In the hospital or birthing center by now, the flurry of activity may have robbed you of your ability to focus. While your cervix is dilating from five to eight centimeters, you may be put through the rigors of being checked in, changing into a hospital gown or preferably your own comfortable labor T-shirt or gown, and having the nurse or technician take your blood pressure and pulse. An internal exam will alert everyone to the baby's progress. You may also be asked to provide a urine sample that will show any traces of sugar and protein. The baby's position will be checked manually by a nurse or midwife who will feel your abdomen. An obstetric stethoscope will be used to listen to the baby's heartbeat and you may be hooked up, at least temporarily, to a fetal monitor. The monitor will reassure you that the baby is getting enough oxygen and is able to handle the contractions. If you aren't confined to bed and can stay up and about, ask if you can take a shower. The warm water will calm you and, if you've been sweating through the trip to the hospital or during prior contractions, your skin will feel clean and cool.

- Your journey through this active labor stage may take two to three hours. This is so highly variable that I hesitate to even highlight the time. However, having a gauge of your progress can be so helpful and comforting. At least you know that it's not going to last forever. When you spend time in active labor, you can certainly lose your sense of optimism.
- Your cervix has dilated more than four centimeters and you need to reach ten. Your contractions are coming closer together regularly, as close as three to five minutes apart, and they can be intense, lasting forty-five seconds. These strong contractions are dilating your cervix. Don't pay any attention to nurses, interns, or even your doctor if your dilation is slower than you want. Some women seem to stay at one spot for hours and then suddenly jump to ten centimeters. Others make steadier progress and reach the same point. Every labor is different. Just keep your attention focused on riding the waves of your own. Occasionally an insensitive aide or obstetrician may mention that you are only five or six centimeters dilated with a long way to go. The frustration and depression about your labor's speed can make you feel even more miserable than you may already be. During active labor, your stage of childbirth can change very quickly, so dismiss bad news or predictions of how much longer you'll have to spend in hard labor.
- Your membranes may rupture now. If the amniotic sac hasn't already broken, it will now or very soon.

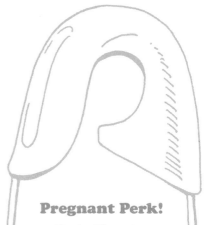

- You could notice bleeding from your vagina. Don't let this blood frighten you. It's normal and often is just more bloody show being expelled.
- Your face may turn red and you'll feel flushed and perhaps panicky. Your uterus is really working intensely hard and needs lots of oxygen. Try panting or using short, speeded-up breaths as the contraction peaks. Take a deeper, cleansing breath and then blow out air as it ends.
- You could be very thirsty. You are moving into what is often considered to be the hardest stage of labor known as *transition*. Your cervix is trying to dilate those last two or three centimeters, from seven or eight up to ten. Ask for ice chips, a lollipop, or something to suck on. Don't take no for an answer because you definitely need to be hydrated for the road ahead.
- Your backache could be intense. The baby's head is pushing on your backbone. Have someone massage your lower back. It won't last long.
- The muscles in your legs could cramp up. If your legs start to shake, have your partner hold them still and flex your feet up and down. Put on socks.
- You could feel tired and ready to call it quits. Concentrate on breathing slowly, easily, and alongside each contraction. Get up and walk around even if someone has to hold you up or if you need to lean back on a wall for support. Change positions. Ask for pain relief. Don't hold yourself to some previously set standard of behavior. You've never done anything like this before if this is your first birth. You are running an incredible race toward childbirth.

Transition

Here's the part where you want to growl at your loving mate, kill the doctor, hurl negatives at the nursing staff, and generally give up the whole notion of becoming a mother. As your cervix dilates the last distance to full opening, your body feels pretty wrecked. You lose track of your old self. I can recall being totally out of it and unable to focus on the poster of waves crashing onto the pretty

Pregnant Perk!

Think of Something Wonderful

Picture yourself in a pleasant place. Make a mental image of it. Perhaps a calm lake or mountain view will put your mind at rest. Visualize this scene on purpose as you slowly let each part of your body go limp. Breathe deeply. Aim for at least ten minutes or longer if you can. Warm hands mean a relaxed body. If your hands are still cool, you know you are still tense. Put them on your neck to test the temperature. Stay put until they warm up.

beach I had propped against the wall opposite my hospital bed. In fact, I was under the waves and in fear of drowning. Rest assured that transition is relatively brief and probably won't last longer than an hour.

- You could be nauseous and may even vomit.
- You may get the shivers and shakes.
- Your back could be killing you.
- Contractions are right on top of each other, barely minutes apart and each lasting a minute. Because it can be nearly impossible for you to keep your thinking straight, a clear-headed partner can come in very handy now. Someone should be wiping your forehead with a cool cloth, breathing in synch with every breath you take, and helping you emotionally with words of comfort. What you need to hear are words like: "You can do this. I know you can. Just a few more moments. That's all it takes. I'll get the doctor. You are almost there." In the meantime, use short little panting breaths when you are on top of the contractions and especially if you feel the urge to push and have been told to hold back.
- You could feel pressure in your rectum. That's your baby.
- Hiccups, twitching legs, and absolute exhaustion. Move around if you can. Change your positions. Have someone massage your legs.
- You may be either too hot or too cold. Ask for a cool cloth to be placed on your forehead or around the back of your neck if you are warm and sweaty. If you are too cold, put on warm socks and wrap a soft cover around your shoulders. These chills, shakes, and sweats indicate your body is in the midst of the worst phase. The only good part about it is that you are almost to the point of pushing out your baby.
- Falling asleep in mini-seconds is possible.
- You may feel like pushing even though your cervix hasn't reached full dilation.

Resist the urge to push until the doctor or midwife gives you the go-ahead. Although your body may be demanding that you push, if your cervix isn't open, you'll end up pressuring your baby's deeply engaged head up against an unopen passage. Pant. Blow out. Remember that this is only momentary and that urge to push is signaling an ending in sight to the toughest part of labor.

Second Stage

The Pushing Part

Hold on. Childbirth educator Rebecca Rowe Parfitt once stated that this effort, forcing your baby out into the world in a normal, vaginal delivery, "is like pushing a grand piano across a large warehouse floor alone."

- Your cervix is finally opened to approximately ten centimeters and the urge to push can be overwhelming. Thank goodness you have the green light to start pushing along with each contraction because as much as this part can hurt, it is also more rewarding. This second stage can last from forty-five minutes up to, or beyond, two hours, especially if this is your first baby. For second-time births, pushing can be shorter work. If you aren't scheduled to deliver right in your labor room, then this is the point when hospital personnel may choose to move you to the delivery room.

  Good news: The contractions still arrive regularly—every two to five minutes—and can be really strong, but because they aren't quite as close together, a bit of breathing room in between will feel heaven-sent. You'll have a chance to rest and may want to change positions. Pushing is very hard work, but the pain may change from the intense gripping you've experienced to more of a stinging sensation. You may also be more alert now, having made it through transition.

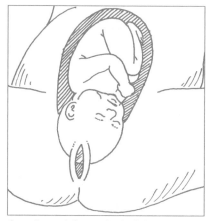

Once the cervix is completely dialated, the baby begins to move down the birth canal.

Some pushing tips:

- Find a position where you will work with gravity, not against it. Can you kneel up on the delivery table and put your arms around the supportive shoulders of two people on either

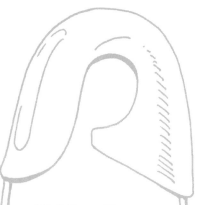

Waiting Games

"She awakened Frank and described the pain, the nausea. The Lamaze class had prepared her for the procedure that would follow if this was really labor. But she could not say for sure that it was. She had suffered no sickness, no pain, for the first eight and a half months of her pregnancy. So this must be labor. On the other hand, she was not feeling regular contractions, her water hadn't broken, and she had no vaginal bleeding. She made coffee. Frank put a roll of dimes in his pants pocket for phone calls, in case they went to the hospital. They sat in the dinette to wait. . . . They waited for fourteen days."

—Sandra Sohn Jaffe and Jack Viertel, *Becoming Parents*, excerpted in *New Mother News*

side? Try sitting up, propped by pillows, with your legs apart, and grip the back of your knees. Put your chin down. If you are in a birthing room and not confined to bed, try squatting. If squatting unsupported is too difficult on your legs, try leaning back against a chair while someone holds your shoulders. Your knees should be spread apart so the full pressure of the baby's head is right on your perineum.

- Give yourself a few contractions to synchronize your pushing efforts. The obstetrician, nurse, midwife, or your partner should start giving you signals on when to push for maximum effect: at the peak of the contraction. This part of delivery goes faster if you give it every ounce of energy left in your body . . . at the right moments. You may be asked to stop pushing, for instance, as the baby's head is ready to emerge. You could be asked to pant or take shallow breaths to prevent your skin from tearing. However, keep in mind that your vaginal tissues are extraordinarily elastic.

- Throw your embarrassment and caution to the wind. Your obstetrician and the other people at your side, including your mate or significant other, aren't there to judge the state of your bodily functions. Seriously, most of them have seen just about "everything" when it comes to childbirth. Don't be concerned about your backside hanging out or any urine or leftover fecal matter that may be eliminated at this late stage. This is natural. Keep your mind focused on the baby whose head is probably within view of everyone in the room with you. This emergence of the head at your vaginal opening starts with a small patch of skin visible during the peak of a push. The patch may recede when you rest but will reappear at the next contraction. Life gets exciting for everyone. The end is near. Put your hand down to feel your baby during hard pushing. That first touch may be just what you need to keep on pushing. You might want to ask for a mirror to see your baby being born.

- Relax your legs, pelvic area, and especially your backside in between pushes. It's only natural to tense up, especially if you didn't receive an epidural.

- Push down smoothly and hold your breath as you bear down. Grunt if you must, but don't let frustration or fear stop you from going with your natural inclination to push.
- Take deep, calm gulps of air, and close your eyes after a contraction.

The Best Part: Birth

- The head crowns. This happy ending to labor and delivery can almost come as a quick surprise after all your hard work. Unless your baby is arriving in a breech position, the head will finally bulge right out of your vaginal opening in what is called *crowning*. You may be asked to stop pushing for a moment, which will seem quite impossible. Give it your best shot, however. Follow instructions on when to push and when to hold up. What you are doing is protecting the baby's head and your own perineal skin.

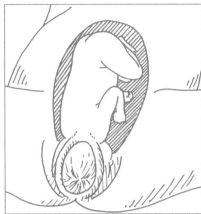
Crowning occurs when the top of the head is visible.

- Your vagina stings. Not really pain but certainly not pleasant, the sensation is caused by your overstretched skin. The obstetrician or midwife may decide on an episiotomy if your skin doesn't appear to be willing to stretch another single millimeter. Massaging the shiny, thin tissue may also be an option now to eliminate the need for cutting or tearing. The stinging only lasts for a few seconds and can be followed by numbness. After all that you've been through, this natural numbing is not such an awful side effect.
- The head comes out under the control of the practitioner. If the head is released too rapidly, tears in the covering of the brain can result. After a series of frustrating pushes forward followed by retreats, the head ordinarily comes first, with the chin facing downward. You may feel a gush, a pop, or a slippery sensation, unlike most anything you've ever experienced. Even as the head is the only part of the body born, your birth attendant will gently search for the umbilical cord to make sure it hasn't become wrapped or tangled dangerously around the baby's neck. Quickly, as you keep pushing, the head will turn to one side, leaning toward the shoulders.

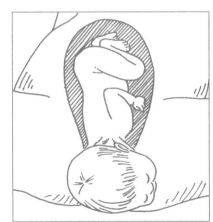
Once the head is completely visible, the doctor will help position the baby so that it's head is in line with its shoulders.

The doctor may wipe the eyes, nose, and mouth and suck any mucus or fluid from her upper respiratory tract using a little bulb syringe.

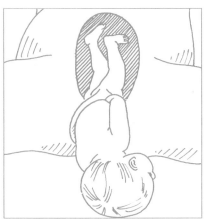

The rest of the body easily slides out, and the birth is complete.

- The rest of the body slides out. Amazed and possibly tearful, you may feel overwhelmed on all fronts at this point. Is it a boy or a girl? Is your baby all right? So much is happening and you may be so exhausted that your reactions are unpredictable. Some babies actually cry out with that first breath just as they are caught coming into the world. Others take a second to orient themselves to the strange, bright, cooler environment. Keep in mind that your womb was at body temperature and watery. Imagine the shock if you can. Wouldn't you cry about such a rapid climactic change? The shock to the baby's respiratory system can jumpstart breathing immediately. The obstetrician usually lifts the baby up and while still connected to you by the umbilical cord, places him or her on your stomach. My son Zach quickly urinated straight up into the air and brought on waves of laughter from everyone in the delivery room, including me.

- The cord is cut. Leaving the placenta still inside your uterus, the cord that connected you to the baby will be clamped and then cut. It may pulse with blood flow for a few minutes and some experts suspect that waiting until the baby is breathing easily is a good idea before severing the connection. However, if the cord is too tight, too short, or endangering the baby in any way, it will be cut quickly. You or your partner may be given the option of doing the cutting yourselves, in fact. If you are squeamish about this, don't feel guilty about saying no thanks. However, consider that it is an opportunity of a lifetime and that doctor or midwife will show you exactly what to do. Now, having made this recommendation, I must admit that my husband fainted when offered the instrument to cut me free from our daughter, Maggie. Exhausted, excited, amazed by the emergence of his second child, he claims that he had no control. A quick whiff of smelling salts brought him back to our sides.

The Third Stage

Pushing the Placenta Out

Your uterus continues to contract as long as the placenta remains inside. Attached to the endometrial lining, the placenta is bloody, soft, and weighs about a pound. The doctor may press down on your abdomen, massaging your uterus to help nudge this third-stage process along. You could also be given a little synthetic hormone to keep your contractions coming and rid your body of the last vestiges of the pregnancy. A gentle tug on the end of the cord, which is hanging free at your vaginal opening, may also be tried to loosen the placenta. You'll be asked to push even though your attentions are certainly elsewhere now. It's important to expel all parts of the placenta because even a tiny remnant can cause bleeding and problems for you later.

Still in the Grips of Delivery Shock

In some hospitals the baby is moved to a warm incubator nearby. Or your mate could be having the pleasure of waltzing around the room with the new person in your family.

- You may be so tired you can hardly keep your eyes open.
- You could get the shakes or chills. Ask for a blanket. Let people know how cold you are.
- You'll have a bloody vaginal discharge called *lochia*. Similar to a heavy menstrual period, lochia may last for several weeks.
- You may need to have stitches to repair any tearing or the episiotomy if you had one. If you haven't had any anesthesia up until now, a local may be administered to take the ouch out of the stitches needed to sew up such a sensitive area.
- Your emotions could swing wildly. You don't have as much control as you want. You may experience exhilaration, shock, anger (about not realizing how hard it was going to be), joy (because it was so easy and you expected the worst), or feel unconnected to the real world, including your baby (normal, don't worry), proud, and amazed at the baby you were able to create.

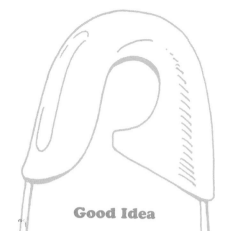

Good Idea

If you are going to breastfeed, ask if you can begin as soon as the baby is born. A sucking infant can start a chain of hormonal reactions that actually help expel the placenta. The sucking stimulates your uterus to continue its muscular contractions and also seems to inhibit blood flow inside your bruised gynecological tract. Even if you feel silly or scared about the whole breast-feeding adventure, take the baby and let him or her rest against your breast. This amazing human touch may help you stand the let-down or any painful aftereffects of the birth.

- You'll be cleaned up perhaps at the same time as your baby is dried, rubbed down, measured, weighed, tested, foot-, and fingerprinted. A sponge bath to your lower body will feel just wonderful now. The doctor may also check your vagina to make sure blood clots have been expelled. Someone will help you into a clean hospital gown and a sanitary napkin.
- Ask for something to drink and a few minutes to bask in the glow of your success. As your head clears and your body settles into a slower rhythm, make sure to take the time to hold your baby, have a picture taken, and kiss your mate. If your baby is healthy and not in need of extra medical care, these few moments can be priceless. Look into each other's eyes. Breathe deeply and force yourself to smile. If you do not feel a wave of instantaneous motherly love, don't feel guilty. Even with eyes at half mast, anger at what you may or may not have expected about the birth, frustration about the hospital or any delivery room procedures that irked you, you are still creating a happy memory.
- You may be whisked off to a recovery room. Ask to have your baby with you for the next hour or so. Open your champagne or sparkling fruit juice. Don't anticipate anything. Simply live in the moment. If you delivered in a birthing room, you'll probably stay put for a little while, if not for your entire recovery period. The bottom half of the bed, which was detached for the birth, can be hooked up once again so you and your celebrating visitors are more comfortable.

C-Section Delivery

The word *cesarean*, sometimes spelled *caesarean*, may come from the Latin verb, *caedere* which means "to cut," and Julius Caesar himself may or may not have arrived in this world after a surgical birth. If you end up having a cesarean, or more commonly known as a C-section, you can rest assured that something warranted this abdominal delivery. Don't feel guilty or angry. Even anthropologist Margaret Mead once wrote that "All of the complicated kinds of equipment that we have developed for childbirth have been developed with some kind of reason originally. There are cases where childbirth is surgery. And this of course is the question of a Caesarean. This is surgery, it is good surgery, it saves the baby who might otherwise have died."

C-sections can be scheduled months or weeks in advance, performed after labor has begun, or under serious emergency conditions to save you or your baby's life. Why a C-section?

- The baby's head may be too large to fit through your pelvis in a condition known technically as *cephalopelvic disproportion*.
- Fetal distress caused by any number of conditions, including an umbilical cord wrapped around the neck
- Problems with the placenta
- Abnormal presentation of the baby coming down the birth canal. For instance, if your baby is arriving feet first, then a C-section could be a wise decision.
- You have diabetes, toxemia, or preeclampsia
- Prolonged, going-nowhere-fast labor
- Previous C-section deliveries
- You are expecting more than one child

What to Expect During a C-Section

If you have any advance warning about your C-section, you'll probably be offered an epidural or spinal anesthesia. Your mate may also be allowed to stand by you and ready to hold the baby. If it's an emergency, things could move quickly and you'll have fewer options. You may also be given a general anesthetic that will make you unconscious, but that is not always the case. Most dads are asked to step outside when general anesthesia has been administered, but you might want to talk to your doctor about special circumstances during childbirth.

- You'll be hooked up to an intravenous needle in your arm to receive fluids as well as pain medication. Ask to speak to your anesthesiologist. Just say hello and ask him or her what kind of pain medication you'll be having.
- Your pubic hair will be shaved either completely or just along the top where the incision will be made.

- You will have a catheter inserted into your bladder. Because your bladder is located right in the middle of all the surgical action, the doctor will want to make sure it stays small, out of the way and, therefore, empty.
- In the operating room, a surgical curtain will be dropped just at your chest. To spare you the close-up encounter with an incision into your own abdomen. By the way, you may hear the action if you've had an epidural and you could also experience a strange, zipped-open sensation as the incisions are made to the outer layer of your skin and then the uterus itself.

  There are two types of cuts the obstetrician can choose. The most popular is the bikini, or *transverse*, cut, which is made just above the natural line of your pubic bone and less than six inches long. Bikini cuts heal nicely and become nearly invisible once your pubic hair grows back. A vertical cut can also be made and would extend straight up from your pubic area for several inches. Keep in mind that this outer cut may not correspond to the actual slit the obstetrician will make into your uterus inside. A cut to the lower end of the womb, where the uterus is thicker, is considered the safest option because it causes less bleeding. Ask your doctor what kind of incisions were made inside your uterus. There are circumstances under which he or she may be forced to cut in a different direction once inside, but you'll want to know where your scars are to anticipate future hot spots in your health. For example, the classical or old-fashioned vertical incision, which is made at the top of the uterus, may prohibit you from having future vaginal deliveries.
- The baby's head will be lifted out first. Sucked from his watery environment, your newborn ought to look less stressed, bruised, beaten, or under the weather if the C-section took place before labor began. Mucus may be sucked from his nose and mouth even before the rest of the body is pulled out. You may hear a whooshing sound as the amniotic fluid is vacuumed out.

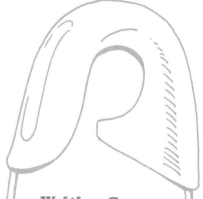

- From beginning to end, you could spend forty-five minutes in the OR.
- Hold your baby or have your mate do so, while you are being stitched closed.
- Recovery can be a bit more complicated than for a vaginal delivery. You've had major abdominal surgery, so don't let anyone try to fool you into thinking otherwise. Your incision is going to be painful and may make it difficult for you to hold your baby or begin breastfeeding. Ask for pain relief. If you are prone to stomach upsets, tell your doctor ahead of time. You don't want to start throwing up and tear out stitches, so preventive measures may be in order.
- Get up and out of bed because movement will help your digestive tract back into action. You could have gas pains. When you laugh, sneeze, or cough, hold onto your incision with both hands. Stitches, if they aren't the dissolvable kind, may remain in place for several days. Gentle exercise is going to help you find your stomach muscles again and so will taking it easy, too. Although it may sound like an impossible prescription, take it easy for at least six weeks. Yes, I know you have a new baby, but learn how to ask for help and don't plan any major events or parties for the immediate future. If you have other children at home, hire regular sitters or arrange to trade future time with other moms. Yes, you will feel better—and sooner than you think!

Vaginal Birth After a C-Section?

Years ago, having one cesarean section automatically meant that any future babies would be born by C-section as well. This is no longer the case. A vaginal delivery is safer, the recovery period is shorter, and doctors now realize that if the first incision was made to the lower, stronger portion of the uterus, then you may be able to sidestep future C-sections. The benefits of a vaginal birth outweigh the risks of a cesarean.

Waiting Games

"Enlightened doctors in the Solomon Islands of the South Pacific believe they have the ideal method for coaxing out reluctant newborns. It is said that when a woman is late giving birth, natives take the father down to the low tide mark and tie him to a stake. At the same time, the mother-to-be is taken to an over-hanging bluff to watch the tide come in.

"The idea is that she will force herself into final labor before her husband drowns at high tide. According to reports from the South Pacific, they haven't lost a father yet."

—Morton Walker, D.P.M., Bernice Yoffee, R.N., and Parker Gray, M.D., *The Complete Book of Birth*, excerpted in *New Mother News*

I Was Wondering . . .

I've heard that labor and delivery room nurses can range from saints to sinners straight from a Stephen King novel. Is there anything I can do in advance to make sure the people who are by my side are actually on my side?

Yes, stories about nurses' bedside manners can frighten you. When you are pregnant, your focus on professional care centers on your practitioner and the setting where you will deliver your baby. You may not even consider the fact that once you enter the hospital or birthing center, you'll be spending most of your time with the nursing staff, not your practitioner. If you have opted for a midwife, you may see more of him or her, but nurses will still be critical to your birth experience. Almost all labor and obstetrical nurses are women who work hard and want to help you. Of course, what you want from them is support, information, enthusiasm, positive feed-back, and lots of tender, loving care. Negative comments or criticism are not going to help you. Above all, you want the nursing staff to be thinking of you and aware of your needs. Even a quick offhand comment can throw your concentration off when you are riding the physical waves of contractions. Keep in mind that, for the nursing staff, a maternity floor can be a magically happy place to work as well as one of high stress and long, exhausting days and nights. Many have received training in all the sophisticated medical practices of birth. Meanwhile, day after day, these nurses must deal with the incredible highs and lows of women becoming new mothers. To you, it's a birth experience of a lifetime. To them, it may be a job. In fact, to save themselves from emotional burnout, some nurses step back emotionally and try not to become involved with laboring women or couples in crisis. Nurses must also bow to the authority of practitioners and specialists who, occasionally, breeze in at the last moment for the delivery while the hard work of labor has gone on for hours beforehand. They carry enormous responsibility but don't always have the authority they might crave. The person who will be key to your experience with the nursing staff is your mate or labor coach. Make certain that you let everyone know that what you need most during the labor, delivery, and birth is praise and support no matter how stressed you become. Negative comments may set you back and if your coach hears one coming, he or she should act like a football player pushing back any offensive tackles. The last thing you need is to be tackled by a snide comment, a rough touch, or indifference. Being aware of the importance of nurses in the birth process can also make the critical difference.

My husband and I have been arguing about whether or not to have our baby son circumcised. We are not bound by any religious convictions, so I'm simply looking for the latest health-related reasons for circumcision. What should we do?

Whether or not to circumcise your new baby boy is highly personal. Technically, circumcision is the removal of the foreskin that covers the head of the penis. A majority of boys are circumcised in the United States in the first days or weeks after birth. Some families do so because of religious custom, while others believe that there are health advantages. A 1989 study by the American Academy of Pediatrics (AAP) found that uncircumcised boys were more likely to develop urinary tract infections. Some parents worry that a child who is not circumcised may be socially hampered living in an environment where most men are circumcised. Meanwhile, other experts caution that there are no medical reasons for circumcision and this practice is a form of mutilation. Talk to each other about the pros and cons and include other family members, friends, or a pediatrician. If you choose to have your baby circumcised, make sure that it's done within days of birth. Don't wait. The procedure takes only minutes to complete but is painful. Ask for a consultation with the doctor who performs the circumcision and be sure to cover all aspects of follow-up care. The penis may bleed, and when you diaper the baby, you'll want to use antibiotic cream or gel and fresh gauze. Done in infancy, the wound heals quickly. However, if your son is premature or at risk in any way, get further medical advice.

Doctor's Note: Circumcision

"First, I believe in circumcision mainly because of the fact that there has never been a malignancy in the penis of a male who was circumcised. Secondly, circumcision doesn't have to be painful because of a cream called Emla, which can be applied to the foreskin to anesthetize it. If a mother and father have decided to have their newborn son circumcised but want to spare him the pain, the hospital nursery should be alerted at least twenty minutes before the surgery so the cream can be applied. It may take up to twenty minutes to numb the foreskin, but there is much less pain for the baby."
—Howard Berk, M.D.

How can I be sure that my baby is all right during labor and delivery?

Your practitioner and the highly trained nursing staff will be watching for signs of fetal distress throughout the birth process. Your vital signs will be closely tracked and all the new obstetrical technology is on your side. The baby's heartbeat may be monitored by a hand-held obstetric stethoscope, the electronic fetal monitor attached to your stomach, or one that may be inserted into your cervix to meet the baby's head. This sophisticated electronic equipment may disturb you, but sometimes the intrusion is exactly what you need to rest assured that everything is proceeding normally. If you are induced, are having an epidural, have a condition that has put you at risk, or your baby has shown any signs of distress during pregnancy, the likelihood of monitoring goes up. Either you or your partner and labor coach should make sure that you let the obstetrical nurse know that you want to be kept informed. Having the medical staff rush around you and not knowing what's happening can be awful. Knowledge is powerful and, while you certainly crave praise and good news about your progress and your baby, you also don't want to be the only person left out of the information loop during childbirth.

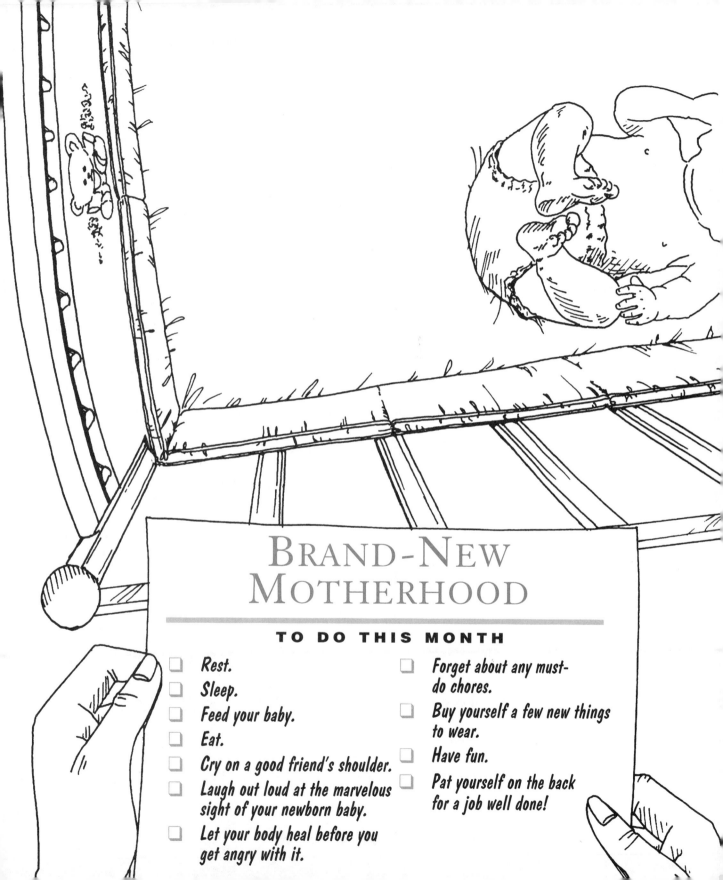

BRAND-NEW MOTHERHOOD

TO DO THIS MONTH

- ☐ Rest.
- ☐ Sleep.
- ☐ Feed your baby.
- ☐ Eat.
- ☐ Cry on a good friend's shoulder.
- ☐ Laugh out loud at the marvelous sight of your newborn baby.
- ☐ Let your body heal before you get angry with it.

- ☐ Forget about any must-do chores.
- ☐ Buy yourself a few new things to wear.
- ☐ Have fun.
- ☐ Pat yourself on the back for a job well done!

When my son Zach was born, he was red-faced with a slight blue body tint. Covered with vernix, that cheesy protective substance his dad likened to cheesecake, he had an elongated head from his trip through the birth canal. Blinded by our emotional high in the delivery room, my husband and I thought he was simply gorgeous. In fact, we believed he was the most beautiful baby in the world. I remember sensing: Could this be real? Examining Zach from toenail tips to his plump baby cheeks and gorgeous dark eyelashes, we were immediately in love. Three years later, when his sister arrived, our emotions ran just as high and love at first sight was just as certain.

Yet, not every brand-new parent feels the tug of mother love so fast and furiously. It definitely isn't even unusual to experience keen disappointment right there in the delivery room. You could feel nothing at all or simply be so darn exhausted that all you want to do is sleep. The reality of the birth experience, the natural physical let-down after what may have been a somewhat grueling ride, bone-weary fatigue, shock about not having a boy or a girl can all cloud your thinking. Even the baby's appearance can make your heart sink. A friend, a perfectly beautiful woman, once related the tale of her own birth. "My father tells me that I wasn't too good-looking. In fact, I looked a bit like Cyclops, with eyes so close-set they looked like one, smack in the middle of my forehead. This surprised my mother, who was assured that because she was having a cesarean delivery her baby would be unsquashed, pink, and beautiful. When I wasn't any of the above, she set out to reassure my bewildered father. 'Don't worry, Ernie,' she said during her brief moment of wakefulness after she'd glimpsed their creation. 'There's always plastic surgery.'"

Don't let first impressions or that first wave of emotions unnerve you. Not only is your own judgment clouded because you may be sweating, leaking, sore, tired, but newborns hardly ever resemble the gorgeous cherubs we see on all those angelic greeting cards and gift book covers. Your baby is a miracle. He can hear, see, smell, cry, coo, and even smile. She can recognize your touch, your voice, and will want to bond with you. Put your baby to your chest. Stare into each other's eyes. Getting to know this strange little creature begins right at birth and is an ongoing physical, emotional complex process.

- If you are going to breastfeed, hold your baby right up against your bare breast. Don't be shy and don't let your feelings of weirdness hamper your natural instinct. Your body isn't producing milk yet, but a substance called *colostrum*. Even a few drops of this liquid helps a newborn's digestive system and will let you get an idea of what "let down" is all about. Milk will start flowing, or "letting down," in two to three days; but your first breast-to-baby encounters help ease you into the process. Massage your nipple and the areola and make sure the baby's mouth is wide open when you insert it. She may not be interested in the least, but your efforts are not in vain.

- Bring up any immediate or dramatic concerns, but rest assured that very few newborns are likely to win any beautiful baby contests. The physical and intellectual changes you'll see in your baby over the next few hours, days, and weeks will soon astound you!

- Ask about the Apgar score. Remember that this quick test is done twice, so the second one is the one you want to remember.

What's Normal in Newborns?

- They lose weight before starting to gain up to an ounce a day. By two weeks, your baby will probably be back up to birth size; and thereafter, she may put on a pound every two weeks. Premature babies sometimes grow a little slower, but most will eventually catch up.

- All five senses are functioning, and your child can see you clearest when you hold him or her seven to ten inches away from your face. Your voice is especially familiar. Researchers say that after only three days, your baby will prefer your voice to a stranger's and any high-pitched voice over lower pitches.

- Muscle control is jerky and usually involuntary. Your newborn arrives with a variety of natural reflexes or involuntary ways of moving. *Grasping* or

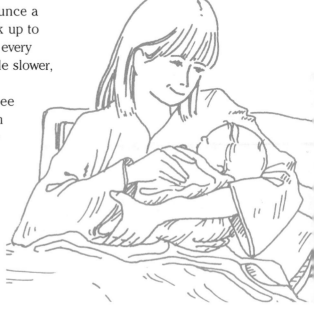

Breast vs. Bottle

Whether to breastfeed or bottle-feed is one of those very personal and yet very complicated decisions for brand-new moms. Pressure from all sides can make you indecisive and anxious. Breast milk meets a newborn's needs perfectly and is digested easily. Yet, formulas are better than ever. Breast milk actually contains substances that can protect your baby from disease until his or her own immune system has matured. However, this is your decision and if you decide to bottle-feed, your baby is not going to suffer. Feeding should be a pleasure, not a challenge. If you are going to breastfeed from a sense of duty or bottle-feed with a sense of guilt, then all the pleasure may be gone. If you think you are leaning toward bottles, however, it's a good idea to put off this decision until after the birth. The colostrum produced by your breasts in the first few days after delivery is wonderful for your newborn. You can always switch to bottles later, but it will be very difficult to start breastfeeding later if your breasts haven't been stimulated to produce milk in those days after childbirth. Whichever method you choose, keep in mind that love, cuddling, and attention are just as critical for your baby as the milk you choose to give him or her.

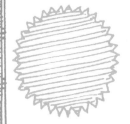

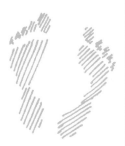

clenching a fist around your finger is one of them. This may be your favorite because it feels like the baby is holding on tightly to you. If you touch his or her lip or cheek, the head will turn automatically toward the touch in what is known as the *rooting reflex*. The *stepping reflex* is fun to try. Hold your baby up so that her feet just barely touch a firm surface. She will look as if she is ready to walk or take little baby steps. When exposed to sudden noises or movements, your baby will exhibit the *startle reflex* by throwing his arms out and crying. As a baby gains more control, these involuntary reflexes gradually disappear.

- Arms and legs usually curl to the chest just as they did in the womb.

- Crying. To communicate, babies must cry. It's okay to pick them up because you can't spoil a newborn. Crying means that your baby needs something: a diaper change, love and attention, to be burped, touched, or fed.

- Sleep-wake schedules are far from predictable. While some experts claim that newborn babies will sleep sixteen hours a day, new parents can often point to much more bizarre schedules. Some sleep in fits and dozes and as little as ten to eleven hours a day, not all of which are at night, unfortunately. Others seem to be unable to keep their eyes open for more than a few minutes at a time. Every newborn is different.

Oh Baby . . . More Little Body Basics

- A strange, pointed, possibly bald head. Caused by the pressure of birth, the head should look normal within two weeks and possibly sooner. On the top is a diamond-shaped area called the *fontanelle* where the bones of the skull have not yet come together. By eighteen months, this soft spot will probably be fused. Although there are no bones there yet, a thick membrane protects your baby's brain. Some newborns have a remarkably thick head of hair while others are quite bald. This state of hairy affairs is also temporary. In fact, some babies lose all their hair, experience a change in color, and grow new soft tufts in the first weeks and months of life.

- Puffy, blue eyes. Your baby's true eye color may not appear until six months into your motherhood experience. The eyelids may be puffed up because of the pressure from those hours in the birth canal. Squinting is quite common. You may even catch a cross-eyed look. What would you be doing if you had spent nine months in a warm, watery, dark womb?

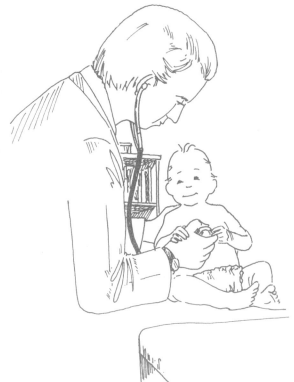

- Funny-looking skin. Spots, rashes, blotches, peeling patches, and red marks caused by the exposure of brand-new, sensitive skin or interventions performed during delivery are common. A baby's skin is immature and not yet ready for prime-time living. Greasy white vernix, as well as a soft furry-like covering of lanugo, or newborn body hair, can also turn you off. Rest assured that the vernix is wiped off right in the delivery room and any noticeable lanugo rubs off within the first one or two weeks. Birthmarks may also be making you wonder. Most of them will vanish soon. Red marks on the eyelids, forehead, and at the very back of the nape of the neck can take up to a year to disappear. Little whitehead pimples are called *milia*, and you may see them around the nose. Caused by oil-secreting glands, the pimples may come and go during the first few days. Strawberry birthmarks can increase in size but may shrink and be gone by age five. If not, modern medicine can do something about them. Blue spots on the buttocks or lower backsides of babies with darker skin are known as *Mongolian spots*. They will fade. If your baby is born with what is known as a *port wine stain*, a bright red or purple mark that is considered to be more permanent, you may relax if you discuss options right away with your pediatrician or family doctor. Most rashes are harmless, but let your doctor know if you want another professional point of view. Also, if you notice red blisters, even tiny ones, which look like bleeding just beneath the surface of the skin, call right away. Known as *petechia*, the pinpoint, purplish-red spots could be a sign of hemorrhage.

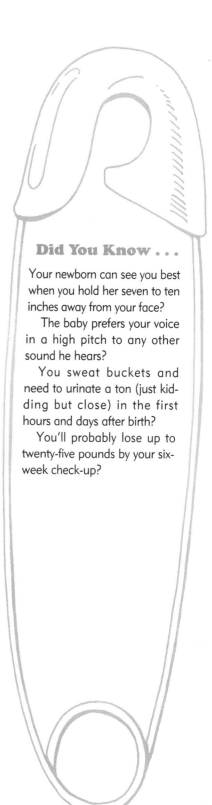

- Leaky, swollen, baby breasts. Your own hormones definitely have an effect on your newborn's little body, so it's quite common for the little breasts of both boys and girls to be swollen and actually leaking a little milk. Don't try to coax any milk out with your fingers and be assured that it will be your own breasts that are swollen and leaking milk very soon. Your baby's breasts will go down within a day or so.

- Oversized genitals. Both newborn boys and girls have genitals that don't quite fit proportionally with the rest of their bodies. Girls may even have a bit of mucus discharge from their vaginas caused by the leftover hormones from you. Boys' testicles can be pulled up into the groin area.

- An umbilical cord stump. A little clamp may remain in place. The cord will fall off within two weeks. In the meantime, ask the nurse or doctor for instructions for keeping it clean and dry.

What Are You Feeling Emotionally?

It rained the entire first two weeks of my son's life. Inside with the baby, I vacillated between states of pure sleep-starved anguish and utter enchantment at what I had created together with my husband. Could this human being actually have come from my body? What a strong personality he had! And weren't new babies supposed to sleep 90 percent of the time? (WRONG!) Shell-shocked, I spent frantic moments rushing through my wardrobe trying to find clothes that would work. Would this shirt unbutton easily for breastfeeding? Would those pants make my overgrown thighs look like two stuffed sausages? But would my old favorite blue-crinkled cotton peasant skirt be better for all those trips to the bathroom? And what was washable? The baby's diapers were dripping onto my lap and I was sweating a lot. My breasts were leaking and they were mountainous. Shirts and tops I had expected to wear had been tried and discarded. Even shoes were problematical because those old reliables—the ones I had worn to the office most days—didn't look or feel right for long days at home. Worse yet, there was simply no time—physically, actually, or emotionally—to shop. A gift certificate from my mother for a small boutique in my neighborhood lay unspent in my

Did You Know . . .

Your newborn can see you best when you hold her seven to ten inches away from your face?

The baby prefers your voice in a high pitch to any other sound he hears?

You sweat buckets and need to urinate a ton (just kidding but close) in the first hours and days after birth?

You'll probably lose up to twenty-five pounds by your six-week check-up?

dresser drawer for weeks and weeks. Amazed at what my body had done, I hated the way it looked.

This period immediately following childbirth may be one of the most wildly emotional times of your life. A variety of outside factors impact almost all new mothers. As Dr. Berk explains, "I feel that postpartum depression is probably stress that occurs to women who have a depressive background. Not every woman who delivers a baby will suffer from postpartum depression, but if the patient has been depressed in the past, is insecure, worried constantly about how to handle the baby, then she may end up with a case of postpartum depression." Suffice it to say that along with your physical upheaval and discomfort, you may feel blue within days after delivery.

- You feel like crying. More than half of all new mothers burst into tears two to three days after giving birth. You are sad, teary, sleep-deprived, not hungry, and unable to make even the simplest decisions.
- You doubt yourself. In your past life, you may have been a pillar of strength, the real navigator in your relationships, but new motherhood has a way of sending you into a tailspin. Is the baby getting enough to eat? Should you take a nap or a shower? Do you need to go to the store or to call your best friend? Indecisiveness is your middle name and you can probably blame much of it on the tailspin new motherhood creates in the wake of childbirth.
- You are angry. Arguing or quietly seething at your husband are common. You have a strong conviction that he is certainly not doing as much as you are and isn't nearly as supportive as he should be under the circumstances.
- You are frustrated that a little baby can take up so much energy and time. The reality of caring for a newborn twenty-four hours a day, seven days a week can be a shocker. If the baby is irritable and not as sleepy as the experts had predicted, you may be in even more emotional trouble.
- You feel isolated. If you don't have close family living nearby or other friends who have new babies, you can be left on your own more than ever before in your life. Confronted hourly with questions of baby care and issues concerning

your own recovering body, you may see your isolated time stretching forward in miserable directions. What's more, everyone who comes to visit focuses mainly on the baby and not you. After having been the center of attention because of your pregnancy, you are now shoved off to side stage.

- You wonder when your motherly instinct will show up. It takes time to get to know your baby under the best of circumstances and bonding is not always something that takes place immediately.

- You are so proud and happy on some deep level, but you can't imagine why your moods are so miserable. Lack of sound, uninterrupted sleep could be a real factor. Newborn babies have very unpredictable sleep-wake schedules. Your ability to sleep for long stretches will have a direct bearing on your health, mood, behavior, energy, and emotions. Some experts even link your sanity and periods of psychosis to sleep deprivation. Studies have shown that you can go without food for up to three weeks, but if you try the same starvation diet of sleep, you'll go crazy. In fact, a quick comparison of the side effects of sleep deprivation and those of postpartum depression ought to be enough to send all new mothers straight to bed with a prescription for child care. According to National Institute of Mental Health research, if you cheat yourself of sleep you will suffer:

    Lapse of attention
    Inability to respond to critical information
    Slow thinking
    Indecision
    Impaired memory
    Withdrawal
    Erratic behavior
    Weakening of ethical standards
    Irritability
    Unpredictable rages

If your signs of sadness last longer than the initial weeks after birth, ask your doctor about professional help. Brand-new motherhood can be a time of unbelievable stress. Getting some kind of therapy is not just something for you. It's also a gift for your baby.

Good Ideas

- Don't try to be a supermom. Let the crumbs stay on the kitchen floor. Eventually, someone else will do the dirty dishes. Close your eyes to clutter. Focus only on you and your baby. A good rule of thumb is: no housekeeping or cooking until at least two weeks after birth. Not even light chores should be on your list right now. Be a slug or couch potato.

- Find another new mother you can speak with regularly or perhaps even every day. I had a friend with whom I could cry about not being able to get a shower. We would laugh about still being in our pajamas at 3 P.M. on some days. Small victories are the name of your new game.

- Take a walk alone. Even if you go for only ten minutes at some odd time, you need to clear your head. Walking will also reduce the risk of blood clots, and if you've had a C-section, the gas and indigestion will be away sooner.

- Consider mini-vacations that will pep you up. Can you schedule a lunch date? Order a new outfit from a mail-order catalog? Rent a romantic movie to watch in the middle of the afternoon when you are feeding the baby? These personal treats are not a sign of your selfishness. If you don't take care of yourself first, you won't be able to take care of the baby.

- Nap often and every time your baby is quiet. Even if you suspect that you can't sleep, simply lie down and let your sore, tired body sink into a bed. A couch will not do. Put yourself on a bed.

- Investigate exercise classes for new mothers, but don't even consider strenuous routines. If you delivered vaginally, you may have been advised to start simple exercises like the Kegels, which will help bring back the muscle tone to your bladder. According to Dr. Philippe Zimmern of the University of Texas Southwestern Medical Center, "The benefits of pelvic muscle or Kegel exercises last a lifetime." Women are more likely than men to suffer from urinary incontinence, so anything you have done during pregnancy or can do right away in this brand-new motherhood state is preventive. Make them part of your daily routine. Try to control the vaginal and anal sphincter muscles every time you urinate. Stop your flow in midstream and hold it for at least five to ten seconds. Relax. Zimmern recommends these little secret moves be done anywhere from thirty to eighty times a day.

- Try lying on your back and raising your chin to your chest. Add a few modified leg lifts to start tightening your abdominal muscles, but don't expect too much. The joints in your body are all still very loose. Any routine that involves running, jumping, knee-bending, squatting, or sudden shifts in body weight is not recommended. If you are a C-section mom, wait and ask your doctor for any precautions.

- When someone asks, "Can I help?" be prepared to explain just where you need assistance. Don't be polite. Assume that this person really does want to pitch in. Put things like kitchen chores and laundry on the top of your list because you may be overwhelmed by the way the dirty clothes' hamper fills up so fast.

Let's Get Physical

Giving birth may be the hardest physical work you'll ever perform. They don't call it *labor* lightly. As a brand-new mom, you need lots of sleep, good food, quiet unpressured periods of time to see and touch your baby, and lots of support. Sound impossible? Try to make these ingredients come together so you can enjoy being a mother. If you are tired, stressed, hungry, angry, or upset, then it will be nigh impossible to see this new role as anything but a burden.

A Few Body Basics

In the hours and days after childbirth, your postpartum body takes a tumultuous ride back nearly to its prepregnant state. In any other situation, the changes would constitute a life-threatening cascade. Author Debra Insel put it so perfectly when she wrote, "I got quite grossed out by all of the blood. All of a sudden the messiness of the birth, the continual bleeding afterwards, the dripping of my breasts, not having good control of my kegel muscles (floor of the pelvis muscles) just disgusted me. Here was a biologist who, in fact, had been fascinated with all the biological process, and I did not even look at the placenta." Rest assured that if other women can get through this new mother mania, then so can you. Here are other normal side effects you may experience:

- You may have cramps. While the uterus tries to contract back to its prepregnant state, it actually keeps on contracting. You can feel these contractions called *afterpains* as cramps for several days. Nursing moms are even more acutely aware of the contractions as they begin to breastfeed. The top of your uterus, which you may even be able to feel through your abdomen, is up around your belly button right after childbirth. Within ten days, it shrinks all the way back down to the level of your pubic bone or one-twentieth the size it was at the beginning of labor. Give your uterus three cheers for such a monumental undertaking, and if the pains become severe, ask your doctor, the nurse, or midwife for a recommendation or prescription for a mild painkiller.
- You'll have bloody discharge. Bleeding from your vagina is normal for at least six weeks or even beyond. All the excess

bulk from your shrinking uterus has to go somewhere and it is expelled from your body as *lochia*, another word for discharge. Your flow will be heavy at first and bright red with big clots, and you'll need a supply of sanitary napkins because tampons are not advised because of the risk of infection. The color may gradually change to pink and then yellow or brown and the flow will taper off within ten to fourteen days. However, the bright red color may begin again at times, especially after breastfeeding. You could pass clots and tissue as this material is sloughed off and your body heals. Speak with your doctor about any aspect that worries you, and check before taking medication. Breastfeeding, in fact, can slow the flow as well as a shot of oxytocin following delivery. Take it easy. Strenuous activity is not going to help your uterus recover.

- Your cervix begins to heal. While your uterus shrinks up, your cervix builds back up. Within ten to fourteen days, the cervix closes up the opening to your uterus.

- Your perineal area is sore. That area between your vagina and rectum, whether you've had stitches or not, can take weeks to recover. Hemorrhoids make this healing time more excruciating. Use ice packs to reduce swelling. Keep a plastic squirt bottle filled with warm water (a "peri bottle") next to your toilet so you can douse yourself whenever you are in the bathroom. Dry heat from your hair dryer or a heat lamp can feel nice. Don't get close enough to burn yourself, however. Take sitz baths. Fill your tub with just a few inches of warm water and sit down. When you lie down, stay on your side and put a pillow under your bottom. Buy a plastic hemorrhoid ring to sit on. You can find them at most drugstores.

- Your vagina doesn't seem the same. The skin of your vagina, which is very elastic and has numerous folds, remains smooth and stretched for up to three weeks. Gradually, you'll start to see it return to gain the normal folds and creases. However, some moms note that their vaginas are never quite the same. Everyone is different. Some say that they are actually more sensitive, others report being less so and having a different shape.

- Urinating is painful. Your bladder can be very sore indeed from the trauma. Pushed out of shape and swollen, the structures of the bladder take time to get better and back to normal. You may even have a bout of urinary tract infection. In the meantime, every trip to the bathroom can be something to dread. It hurts and you may sense a tingling, too. What can compound the situation is your need to go almost as often as you did when you were pregnant as your body sheds excess fluid. Take a long shower as soon as you feel strong enough and let the warm water relax your muscles. Let the water run over your sore bottom and urinate right there in the shower. If you are dealing with stitches from an episiotomy, the warm flow is a great idea.

- Your bowels may seem to be "paralyzed." Millions of brand-new moms suffer from constipation. Where it was just recently cramped, your bowel is now floating in lots of space and has lost any tightness or tone it once had. Your abdominal muscles, so critical to pushing forth a bowel movement, are probably nearly zilch, too. Yet, doctors, nurses, and midwives all urge you to try having a bowel movement within a day or two after delivery to make sure everything works. Drink lots of water. Move around. Eat high-fiber foods. Realize that you are normal. Torn between the fear of going and the real urge to go, you can also ask about recommendations for a stool softener or a laxative. If you are breastfeeding, check with your practitioner before taking any medication. When you do feel like you must go, try holding a clean sanitary pad up against any sutures or stitches while you empty your bowel. Sounds a little tricky, of course, but if you are afraid of ripping open any stitched areas, the sanitary pad will give you confidence.

- You sweat buckets. In the first week after birth, you may find yourself sweating profusely even when the air temperature is quite cool and anything but humid. What's happening is that your body has to reduce the volume of blood it pumped up to accommodate the baby. You can expect to lose up to twenty pounds in a week, in addition to the weight you lost right there

Motherhood Miracle

Pause . . . and Smile

When the baby cries, when you are forced to climb out of bed in the middle of the night yet again, when you find yourself racing from one series of crises to the next, pause for a minute. Force yourself to smile or at least turn off the growl. A constant diet of urgency can make it difficult for you to think clearly. Invest a minute of time in silence, even as life beckons you from every corner, and you may be more effective. Your baby needs such positive pauses as much as you do.

in the delivery room. Such an extreme and physically quick transformation can make you feel not only sweaty but also weak.

- Stitches can be a real, itchy pain in the backside. Most stitches dissolve within a week and external ones may fall out. Pelvic floor exercises can help speed up the healing process. Use ice packs wrapped in soft toweling to soothe irritation and reduce any swelling. Soak in a shallow, warm sitz bath and dry the area thoroughly. Don't stand for an extended time.

- Your breasts will be achy, bulging, and tender. For about two to four days after the birth, your breasts stay pretty much the same as they were at the very end of pregnancy: big but tolerable. Even as you venture into the unknown territory of breastfeeding, what you are really offering your baby at first is colostrum, a pale fluid made up of water, proteins, minerals, and antibodies that will protect the baby until the real milk starts to flow. Then, amazingly, your breasts can become absolutely engorged with milk. Breasts can become so tightly stretched that the baby has a near-impossible time latching on to suck. Because it can take a little time to establish a breastfeeding routine, these days of leaky, engorged breasts can be trying. Don't try to conquer these problems alone. Talk to other nursing moms. If you don't know any, call your obstetrician's office and get advice. This is your body and your discomfort is certainly real. While you are still in the hospital or birthing center, sit down with someone who knows more than you do about lactation. Buy a good book about breastfeeding. (*So That's What They're For: Breast Feeding Basics* by Janet Tamaro is terrific.) Nursing moms can reduce some of the pressure by expressing milk. If you've decided to bottlefeed exclusively, you'll receive instructions about drying up your milk supply. This process may take a few days to accomplish; and in the meantime, you'll be advised to wear an extra-tight bra or perhaps even wrap a towel around your chest. Ice packs and cloths dipped in cool water also help.

Baby Equipment Essentials

Those first few months of new motherhood will go easier if you have the right equipment. Not all of these items need to be purchased. Ask around and you may be able to borrow exactly what you need.

- Baby carrier (Optional but very useful)
- Baby monitor (Optional)
- Backpack (Optional)
- Bassinet or cradle (Optional)
- Booster Seat (Optional but nice to have)
- Bouncing seat (Optional but extremely useful)
- Car seat (Required by law)
- Changing table or dresser/changing table combo (Optional but extremely useful)
- Crib with mattress

- Diaper pail
- High chair
- Jumper (Optional)
- Playpen or porta-crib
- Rocker (Optional but oh so nice)
- Safety gates
- Sling carrier (Optional)
- Stroller
- Swing (Optional)
- Walker/bouncer (Optional)

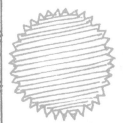
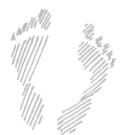

I Was Wondering . . .

**I am scheduled to return to work in three weeks, and
suddenly, I wonder if I've made the right decision. Should
I have requested more time off if possible?**

You have just entered a very special and finite time of your life
called *puerperium*. While it certainly isn't always possible, if time and
finances permit, you should set aside the next six weeks for very personal affairs. The baby needs to learn all about you and you need to
learn how to feed your newborn. Whether you have decided to
bottle-feed or breastfeed, you can't possibly establish any kind of
rational sleeping and eating pattern in three weeks. These tasks you
take on during the puerperium are going to create a definitive wake
in the path of your life as a mother. Don't rush it. Be selfish. Get
acquainted. Sleep. Eat. Be a slug. Let your days dribble away for now.
Forget about being efficient. Take your vitamins. Drink water. (Did you
know that your brain needs water to make all the right chemical con-
nections. If you are dehydrated, you can't think straight at all.) Talk to
other mothers. Kiss your mate. Kiss your baby every time you pick
him or her up. Your sense of time is absolutely out of the ordinary
for now. Don't jump up to rush anywhere. Stop thinking of your time
as scarce because you will make yourself more fragmented than you
may already be. There should be no day in this puerperium stage
that is tightly scheduled. You are in what almost every expert in the
world would describe as a state of turmoil . . . a predictable,
promising, natural outcome to the end of your pregnancy.

**My nipples are so sore that I can hardly stand the pain
when my baby begins to nurse. What can I do?**

Dr. Berk recommends a prescription cream called Masse,
which can be applied to the nipples right after a feeding. Expose
your breasts to the air for ten minutes and then wash them with
warm water before the next feeding. This cream can "help take care
of cracking, sore nipples," says Berk. Ask your practitioner to prescribe Masse.

After every feeding, try vitamin E oil directly on your nipples. Even if the baby must suddenly nurse again, the oil is perfectly safe for the baby. Some moms use petroleum jelly or baby oil, too. Find a private, comfortable place outside and expose your breasts to direct sunlight. Let them "air out" frequently between feedings. Honestly, the soreness will gradually go away as your nipples toughen up. Hang in there. Massage your breasts when you are in the shower but stand with your back to the showerhead. Stay away from soap, which can dry the skin. Always dry thoroughly. A little breastmilk or colostrum rubbed onto your sore nipples can also help. Express some onto clean fingertips and gently apply to your breasts.

My husband is anxious to begin our sex lives, but I'm not sure when that will be possible. This is not a topic I can discuss easily with my obstetrician. What's a good rule of thumb for someone who has delivered vaginally with no problems?

Many doctors recommend that you wait four to six weeks to avoid infection before resuming intercourse, but every couple is different. If your delivery was uncomplicated and you didn't have an episiotomy, then you may want to try sooner. However, your own interest in sex may just not be as keen as your husband's for up to twelve weeks after delivery. Let's face it, if your episiotomy is sore, if your breasts are engorged and leaking milk, if you're trying to feed the baby all day and into the night, if you're tired, if you are constipated, if it burns when you urinate, if you are continually changing sanitary pads because of the continuous bleeding, and if you feel downright alienated from your past life, then sex isn't on your mind. Following a C-section, this four- to six-week time frame before resuming sexual relations is also standard advice. Lack of sleep, feeling unattractive, and the overwhelming responsibilities of baby care really can wreak havoc on what may have been the wildest of libidos. A crying baby is also an immediate turn-off. Talk to your mate about sex and the fact that postpartum symptoms are

Trouble Signs

Call your doctor right away if:

- You run a temperature of more than 100 degrees Fahrenheit. This could mean that you've developed an infection.
- Your discharge changes suddenly to an even brighter red and is nearly unstoppable. A foul smell could also alert you to infection or a piece of the placenta stuck in your uterus.
- A small area in your breasts becomes red or tender. A milk duct could be clogged or infected.
- You have pain in your calf or lower leg. A blood clot may have formed.
- It burns when you urinate. You could have a urinary tract infection.

complicating the issue. Don't let your disinterest and his keen interest in making love become a mountainous issue in the middle of your relationship. Keep the conversation going. The emotional and physical whirlwind of the postpartum period is certainly not a predictor of the rest of your lives together. Even if you don't feel like making love, try to spend quiet, intimate time with your mate. Can you arrange for an at-home "date" when the baby is napping? Cuddle and hold each other. Rest assured that very few couples are able to swing back into an easy sex life immediately after the birth of a baby.

Nothing fits right. Because I'm breastfeeding, some of my tops are just so darn inconvenient, too. Any suggestions?

Your body just doesn't return on a day's notice. No one's does. Even Demi Moore and Madonna didn't have bodies that bounced back the day after childbirth. I know you are probably sick of the sight of maternity clothes by now, but you may need to turn back to that section of your wardrobe for a few weeks. You need clothes that are soft next to your skin and that are easy to get into and out of on all your frequent trips to the bathroom. You are dealing with sanitary pads, a sore bottom, and wobbly thighs, so tight jeans aren't your best bet. Do you have anything with an elasticized or drawstring waist? Skirts are a good idea, but make sure whatever you buy is washable. Consider clothes that are comfortable for napping, too.

In fact, think about your nightgowns or sleepwear. Do you have things in your lingerie drawer that are made of natural fabrics so your skin can breathe better? Stick to cotton or cotton-crotched underpants for your postpartum period. You need more gowns, pajamas, or sleep T-shirts because you may end up changing more than once a night. If you are breastfeeding, ask yourself: Will I be able to have easy access to my breasts in the middle of the night? Will my bare arms get cold on very early winter mornings? Will I be able to pull one arm out and circle up over the baby's body if I decide to nurse in bed? Some gowns are simply too constricting to accomplish this task comfortably. Will the fabric make me sweat even more than I already am? Would I want to be seen wearing this nightgown or pajamas? (Friends, relatives, and neighbors may stop in unexpectedly to see the baby and offer you help.) Last, what will happen when you throw the PJs or gown in the laundry several times a week?

Yes, breastfeeding can make you reexamine your clothes in new and different ways. For six months during the latter part of one of my pregnancies, I would glance longingly at several dresses in my closet. Then, three weeks after the birth, I slipped into one of the looser ones and started to walk out of the bedroom. Then I realized that I would never be able to feed the baby without taking the entire dress off first. There were no buttons, not even a back zipper, and the high neck would have made it impossible to pull down from that direction. I went back and changed to a blouse that buttoned down the front. Later, I realized that even that option required real skill to manipulate. Although buttons-down-the-front may seem to be the best route, think again. Have you ever tried to unbutton a blouse with one hand while cradling a crying baby with the other and trying to appear modest at the same time? You might want to try some soft, loose-fitting turtlenecks or T-shirts or other easily pulled-up tops. There are also special tops just for nursing that you can buy at a maternity store. These have hidden vents and are very easy to use.

Do you have any good advice about nursing bras? I bought several last month, but don't like the way they operate or feel now.

Isn't it amazing how simple little snags can make your life stressful during these first days of motherhood? A bra is nothing to belittle. Get comfortable with this part of the breastfeeding routine right away. Here are some tips: When you shop for a nursing bra, you really need to make sure that you can snap or unsnap, hook or unhook the cup openings with one hand and without looking. You may have your baby in your arms and unhook or snap with one arm under a shirt on occasion. Some nursing bras have built in quick, easy-to-release clasps. Don't be shy about asking a salesperson before you buy new ones. Don't buy nursing bras with plastic cup liners. The plastic is there to protect your clothes from leaky breasts, but it could keep you uncomfortably and dangerously damp. You can always use store-bought nursing pads or even mens' cotton handkerchiefs folded and tucked into your bra cups.

Most brand-new mothers have gone down in chest size but up in bust size. The rib cage actually contracts after delivery even though it doesn't go back to its prepregnant dimensions right away. Your bust, of course, has gone up because of the breast milk your body is producing. For instance, if you wore a 38 C in your ninth month, you may be a 36 D now. Perhaps this size difference is making you uncomfortable. Your bust size is definitely at its biggest during these initial days after childbirth; but after your milk comes in and you and your baby are on a more predictable schedule of feedings, your size will gradually shrink. Nursing bras do come with several rows of hooks or snaps to accommodate your ups and downs. In fact, don't buy a nursing bra with fewer than four adjustments in the back. The hooks or snaps should be at least three or four rows high, too. Bra straps should be wider than the usual three-eighths or five-eighths inch and closer to three-quarters of an inch. This width is especially important for comfortable support if you are a D cup or bigger.

My face looks so tired. Is there anything I can do?

Nervous tension and exhaustion can take a real toll on your face. Sensitive skin, lines under your eyes, oiliness on your nose, dry patches on your cheeks, a strange little rash somewhere else? I know you are incredibly busy and when you aren't you may need to be sleeping, but here are some recommendations worth trying: Stay away from soap. Force yourself to rest. Even short five-minute catnaps can help. Apply an oil-free moisturizer to your face several times a week. Don't pick pimples. Go out into the fresh air. If you are in direct sunlight, use a sunscreen. Drink lots of water.

Why don't my shoes fit anymore?

The hormones that circulated in your pregnant body leave a residual effect that can soften and loosen joints and ligaments for a long time, if not forever. These are the same hormones that allowed your pelvic area to stretch and let your baby emerge, so don't be so hard on your body. Buy new shoes. I used to be a size 7½, but after two children and years of playing tennis, I wear a 9 now. Your feet may need shoes—comfortable ones!—two sizes bigger than those in your closet and under the bed.

I feel so fat. When will I start losing the weight I gained during my pregnancy?

Give yourself time. Most women lose only about ten to twelve pounds at delivery. The rest comes off in dribs and drabs. In fact, don't even get on the scale. Get it out of your sight for now. You really aren't anatomically normal for several weeks after childbirth. It may take you from six months up to a year to coax your body back into shape, but your old size is certainly in reach. Even though your baby, the placenta, and the amniotic fluid are gone, you could weigh as much as you did when you were pregnant . . . for a short time. During the first week, pounds will disappear and this loss should continue for up to ten weeks or more. Most women lose up to twenty-five pounds by their six-week postpartum visit. Even your uterus doesn't automatically shrink back to its normal size, and those abdominal muscles need time and exercise to regain their elasticity.

Give your body a break. Stand up tall. Look for a new outfit that will let you merge your pregnant self into a postpartum period. But most important, feeling badly about your body can actually make you fatter. Sounds absurd, I realize, but it's true. Research has shown that self-esteem can work wonders from the inside out. Fat is certainly more than skin deep. Find something about yourself to love this month. A friend of mine tells me that most women are ashamed of their bodies and dissatisfied with their size. Think curvy for the time being and pat yourself on the back for giving birth to a

The Truth About Getting Back to the Old "You"

You aren't going to be stuck with extra pregnancy pounds forever. Try to look at your new life and begin to create the right balance between calories and exercise. If you are breastfeeding, extra fats and sugars will be stored on your body. You need proteins, vegetables, and carbohydrates to heal and help your baby grow.

The kind of fat you may have gained during pregnancy is not different from any other kind of fat. While you were pregnant, there was an increase in fat production and some new cells may have accumulated around your hips, thighs, and buttocks, as well as any other troublesome spots you are noticing now. This after-the-baby-fat does seem harder to budge at first because all your body's functions, including digestion, have slowed down as a protective measure around delivery time. Don't stay inactive for weeks and weeks now. Get up and get moving to speed up your metabolism and create energy.

Breastfeeding is not going to keep you fatter longer. By producing milk for your baby, you can burn extra calories each day. In fact, brand-new nursing moms may be able to lose weight faster at first. In the meantime, while you continue to breastfeed, you may carry an extra five to seven pounds, which can look like stubborn, ordinary fat cells when you look down at those three numbers on your bathroom scale. However, these pounds are the weight of the milk itself, as well as the glands your body needs to keep on lactating.

Your stomach can get flat again. Your former muscle tone can be regained and even improved. Your abdominal muscles aren't your first priority, however. The vertical muscles in your abdomen may have separated during pregnancy. Don't worry. This condition, called diastasis, is especially common in women who have already given birth. The important thing to remember is to take it easy. Eventually, the separation will heal. However, too much exercise too soon, even mild movements, can exacerbate the situation. In the meantime, ask your practitioner to verify the diastasis and get some expert advice on pulling your abdominal wall back together. Of course, it's okay to start tensing and releasing them, but the real work should be focused on your pelvic floor. Do your Kegels more religiously than any other exercise move now. Save more strenuous workouts for a little later and avoid anything that arches your back or that may stretch out your abdominal muscles too soon. When you walk, make a conscious effort to correct any of the pregnant swagger you may have picked up. Put your shoulders down. Pull in your stomach muscles. Stand up straight and tuck your buttocks under.

new little human being. In the meantime, as Tamara Hill, a mother of five and founder of Fat Chat, based in Augusta, Georgia, says, "Stand up straight. Pull those shoulders back. A confident stature can speak louder than your size. Honestly, good posture can make a profound difference. So just do it."

After a C-section or an unusually complicated deliver, your weight loss may take longer. Increase your vitamin C intake and add some zinc to speed healing. Don't exercise unless your doctor gives you the okay. Your incision must be tightly closed before you even consider getting back into shape. If you have other children at home, losing your pregnancy pounds is also more of an uphill battle, but doable. Start exercising again but take it slowly. Listen to your body. Your activity level undoubtedly dropped in that last trimester, so go slow at first. Tackle some of those prenatal exercises that were recommended because you can increase your muscle tone and strength. A body with muscles burns calories faster and more efficiently than a flabby one. Eat breakfast every day, drink plenty of water, and stay away from junk foods.

I'm not having any fun as a new mother. When will it get easier?

Do something right now to change the way you are looking at your responsibilities. Living in the present is one of the nicest and most important presents you can give to your baby. Kay Willis, founder of Mothers' Matter, a research and support group in New Jersey, and mother of ten, insists that too many modern mothers wish away their children's childhoods waiting for life to get easier. "Having fun is an important parenting skill. If you are constantly anticipating a rosier future, a time when life with your baby will become better than ever, you run the risk of missing the joys of today."

Set aside time for yourself. Everyone needs at least two hours a week to call their own. These hours can't be penciled in for 11 o'clock at night when you are exhausted nor should they be used to do mundane chores. If you can't remember when the last time you had fun was, then you are giving your newborn, as well as your entire family, "leftover" you. Kay says that "Time off from a demanding routine becomes the equivalent of money in your bank account. These are funds you will almost certainly borrow on when life lets you down, and feeling overwhelmed and trapped can make you miserable. You don't teach kids how to be happy. You show them. You are their role model for living happily ever after." So, think about what makes you laugh out loud. Now, don't just think it. Go do it. Forget about the dirty baby laundry, the dishes in the sink, the unmade beds, and the chores on your old to-do list. The most important thing you can do for your baby is to learn how to enjoy mothering.

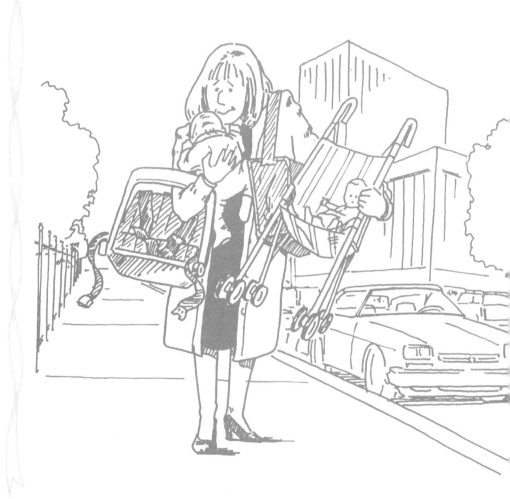

APPENDIX

Organizations and Web Sites That Might Be Helpful

National Organizations

AMEND (Aiding Mothers [and fathers] Experiencing Neonatal
    Death
4324 Berrywick Terrace
St. Louis, MO 63128
Phone: 314-487-7582
Professionally trained lay counselors have experienced the death
of an infant are ready to provide free telephone support.

American College of Obstetricians and Gynecologists (ACOG)
409 Twelfth Street, SW
P.O. Box 96920
Washington, DC 20090-6920
The ACOG Resource Center has wonderful patient education
pamphlets on almost every topic you can imagine dealing with pregnancy. They will mail you up to five different pamphlets. Call the
center at 202-863-2518 between 9 A.M. and 5 P.M. Eastern Standard
Time or fax your questions to 202-484-1595. You can also visit their
Web site at http://www.acog.com. Requests for specific booklets,
which are described in more detail on the Internet, can be e-mailed
to Pamela Van Hine at pvanhine@acog.com.

The American Dietetic Association
216 West Jackson Boulevard
Chicago, IL 60606-6995
Phone: 312-899-0040
Fax: 312-899-1970 (24 hours a day, seven days a week)
Internet address: www.eatright.org
Got questions about eating for two? This is the place to go for
answers.

American Society for Reproductive Medicine (formerly The
American Fertility Society)
1209 Montgomery Highway
Birmingham, AL 35216-2809
Phone: 205-978-5000
Fax: 205-978-5005
Internet address: http://asrm.org
E-mail: asrm@asrm.org
Unable to get pregnant? Contact this group for help and advice
or a referral to a specialist in your area.

ASPO/Lamaze
1200 Nineteenth Street, NW, Suite 300
Washington, DC 20036-2412
Phone: 1-800-368-4404 or 202-857-1128
Internet address: http://www.lamaze-childbirth.com
To find a Lamaze class near you, contact them.

Depression After Delivery
P.O. Box 1282
Morrisville, PA 19067
Phone: 215-295-3994
http://www.behavenet.com/dadinc/
Local support groups meet twice a month. This national organi-
zation functions as a clearinghouse for information and also pub-
lishes a newsletter.

The Institute of Pediatric Nutrition
P.O. Box 2025
Rock Island, IL 61204-2025
Phone: 1-800-721-5BAB (5222)
An organization dedicated to educating parents and professionals
about nutrition for infants and young children, this group can send
you educational materials free of charge.

International Childbirth Education Association (ICEA)
P.O. Box 20048
Minneapolis, MN 55420
Phone: 1-800-624-4934 or 612-854-8660
Fax: 612-854-8772
Internet address: http://www.icea.org
A professional organization, ICEA supports educators, parents, and other healthcare providers who believe in family-centered birth.

La Leche League International
1400 North Meacham Road
P.O. Box 4079
Schaumburg, IL 60173-4048
Phone: 1-800-LALECHE or 847-519-7730 (between 9 A.M. and
    5 P.M. Central Time)
Internet address: http://www.lalecheleague.org
Everything you ever needed to know about breastfeeding.

National Association of Childbearing Centers
3123 Gottshall Road
Perkiomenville, PA 18074-9546
Phone: 215-234-8068
Fax: 215-234-8829
Internet address: http://birthcenters.org
E-mail: ReachNACC@BirthCenters.org
If you are looking for a birthing center in your area, this is the group to contact.

National Perinatal Information Center
One State Street, Suite 102
Providence, RI 02908
Phone: 401-274-0650
Fax: 401-455-0377
Internet address: http://www.npic.org
E-mail: npic@npic.org
Nonprofit center that provides research data on perinatal services, evaluates programs, and checks out hospitals. They offer up-to-date neonatal information.

Postpartum Support, International
927 North Kellogg Avenue
Santa Barbara, CA 93111
Phone: 805-967-7636
Internet address: http://www.iup.edu.an/postpartum
Provides current information on the diagnosis and treatment of postpartum mood and anxiety disorders.

RTS Bereavement Services (formerly known as Resolve Through Sharing)
Gunderson Clinic/Lutheran Hospital
1910 South Avenue
LaCrosse, WI 54601
Phone: 1-800-362-9567 Ext. 4747 (except if you are calling from New York or New Jersey)
NY & NJ Phone: 608-791-4747
RTS provides training and support material for professionals working with parents who have lost a baby through miscarriage, ectopic pregnancy, stillbirth or newborn death. Parents who call will also find a compassionate staff ready to listen and provide resources or referrals to local support groups.

The Triplet Connection
P.O. Box 99571
Stockton, CA 95209
Phone: 209-474-0885
Fax: 209-474-2233
E-mail: triplets@inreach.com
A network of sharing and caring for multiple birth families, this group can provide vital information to expectant parents as well as resources for after the births.

Twin Services
P.O. Box 10066
Berkeley, CA 94709
Phone: 510-524-0863 (Monday through Friday, 10 A.M. to 4 P.M. Pacific time)
E-mail: TwinServices@juno.com
If you know you are going to have twins, contact this group.

Great Web Sites for Pregnancy-Related Issues

BabyCenter
http://www.babycenter.com
"The Web's best for pregnancy and baby"

Caring/Hygeia
An Online Journal for Pregnancy and Neonatal Loss
Using New Technology to Teach Age-Old Feelings and Lessons
The Hygeia Foundation
http://hygeia.org

Parents Place
The Parenting Resource Center on the Web
http://www.parentsplace.com

Parent Soup
http:parentsoup.com

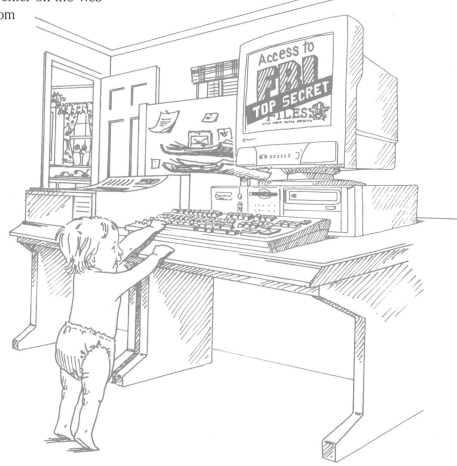

THE

EVERYTHING®

PREGNANCY CALENDAR

The Everything® Pregnancy Calendar

A pregnancy calendar is a handy tool for expecting mothers. Here is one place where you can keep track of your due date, your doctor's appointments, and the changes that are happening with your body. And when the baby arrives, you'll have a wonderful keepsake of each and every day of your pregnancy.

Begin the calendar with the first day of your last period, even if it didn't fall on the first day of the month. Mark it down under the appropriate *day* of the week, (i.e. Wednesday). This is an important date to remember; your doctor will require it to determine your due date. You'll also need the date for your ultrasound appointment, as well as other important tests.

Next, count out forty weeks—or 280 days—from the first day of your last period. This will be your "due date." In most pregnancies it is almost impossible to determine the exact moment of conception, and this is the best way doctors can approximate when you will deliver. Mark this date on the calendar; it should fall on the very last page.

In between, fill out the months and days. While the calendar will look different than a standard calendar, to you it will serve a much more important function. And toward the end of your pregnancy, you'll surely be counting the days until the baby arrives.

Have fun with the calendar, and use it for every aspect of your pregnancy. It can serve as an accessible reminder to know exactly what week you are in, and to keep track of doctor's appointments, scheduled tests, and when to expect their results. Use it as a diary or journal, where you can jot down your thoughts and feelings on particular days that are important to you; the day you first felt the baby kick, the day you stopped feeling queasy, the day your regular clothes stopped fitting, your first shopping trip to the maternity store, the day you somehow "knew" just what the sex of the baby would be. Or anything else that you will want to remember or later share with your new child.

You may want to follow Dr. Berk's advice of weighing yourself only on Friday's, and this calendar can be used as a way to keep track of your weight gain. You can even keep a record of what you've been eating to make sure that you are getting a balanced diet and enough calories as your pregnancy progresses.

One pregnancy legend is that many women deliver on a full moon. You can certainly transfer the lunar cycle from a standard calendar onto this one and see if it will hold true for you!

As you'll hear over and over again, every pregnancy is unique. No two women will have the same calendar, or even use it for the same purposes. If you find this calendar useful, it can become a wonderful momento of this very special time of your life—something that you will cherish for years to come.

Month One _Sept._ (Weeks 1 through 4)

Sunday	Monday	Tuesday	Wednesday	Thursday	Friday	Saturday

Month Two _____ (Weeks 5 through 8)

Sunday	Monday	Tuesday	Wednesday	Thursday	Friday	Saturday

Month Three _____ (Weeks 9 through 12)

Sunday	Monday	Tuesday	Wednesday	Thursday	Friday	Saturday

Month Four

(Weeks 13 through 16)

Sunday	Monday	Tuesday	Wednesday	Thursday	Friday	Saturday

Month Five Feb. _____ (Weeks 17 through 20)

Sunday	Monday	Tuesday	Wednesday	Thursday	Friday	Saturday
	I first felt you move in the morning & a little bit at night!					

Month Six _____ (Weeks 21 through 24)

Sunday	Monday	Tuesday	Wednesday	Thursday	Friday	Saturday

Month Seven _____

(Weeks 25 through 28)

Sunday	Monday	Tuesday	Wednesday	Thursday	Friday	Saturday

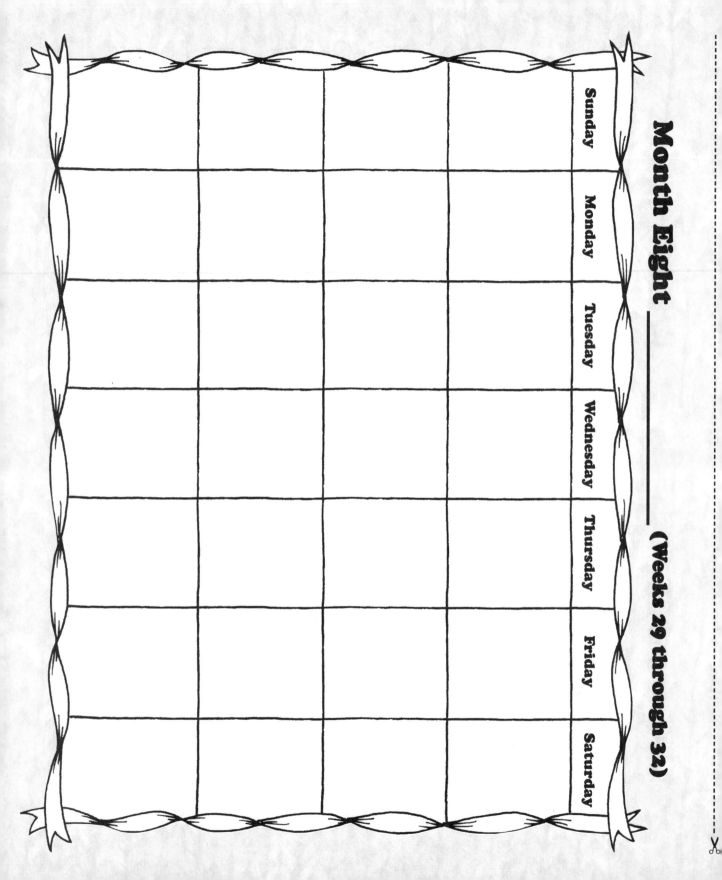

Month Eight

(Weeks 29 through 32)

Sunday	Monday	Tuesday	Wednesday	Thursday	Friday	Saturday

Month Nine
(Weeks 33 through 36)

Sunday	Monday	Tuesday	Wednesday	Thursday	Friday	Saturday

Month Ten _____ (Weeks 37 through 40)

Sunday	Monday	Tuesday	Wednesday	Thursday	Friday	Saturday

Index

EVERYTHING®

The Everything® Pregnancy Organizer
by Marguerite Smolen

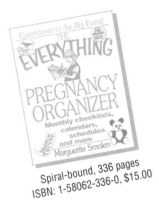

Spiral-bound, 336 pages
ISBN: 1-58062-336-0, $15.00

The Everything® Pregnancy Organizer is a spiral-bound handy planner designed to make the most of these exciting nine months. Arranged in an easy to use month-by-month format, this expectant mother's best friend will help you keep track of doctor's appointments, medical tests, choosing the best name and planning a nursery. Also inside the mother-to-be will find essential medical information on what is happening to the baby's body as well as yours. *The Everything® Pregnancy Organizer* also includes numerous worksheets, checklists and pockets to help you plan and organize these whirlwind months as efficiently as possible.

The Everything® Get Ready For Baby Book
by Katina Z. Jones

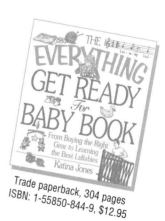

Trade paperback, 304 pages
ISBN: 1-55850-844-9, $12.95

Your baby is coming and you don't know where to begin. You've read the medical texts, you're counting the days, and now you're getting overwhelmed with the never-ending shopping list of "must have" baby stuff. *The Everything® Get Ready For Baby Book* offers tried and true answers to hundreds of your most pressing questions. This comprehensive book focuses on everything you need to do to get ready—the room, your body, and your mind—before the new baby arrives.

Available wherever books are sold.

**For more information, or to order, call 800-872-5627
or visit www.adamsmedia.com**

Adams Media Corporation, 260 Center Street, Holbrook, MA 02343

We Have EVERYTHING

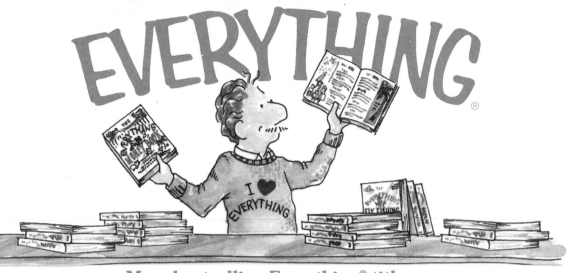

More bestselling Everything® titles available from your local bookseller:

Everything® **After College Book**
Everything® **Astrology Book**
Everything® **Baby Names Book**
Everything® **Bartender's Book**
Everything® **Bedtime Story Book**
Everything® **Beer Book**
Everything® **Bicycle Book**
Everything® **Bird Book**
Everything® **Casino Gambling Book**
Everything® **Cat Book**
Everything® **Christmas Book**
Everything® **College Survival Book**
Everything® **Crossword and Puzzle Book**
Everything® **Dessert Book**
Everything® **Dog Book**
Everything® **Dreams Book**
Everything® **Etiquette Book**
Everything® **Family Tree Book**
Everything® **Fly-Fishing Book**
Everything® **Games Book**

Everything® **Get Ready For Baby Book**
Everything® **Golf Book**
Everything® **Guide to Walt Disney World®, Universal Studios®, and Greater Orlando**
Everything® **Home Buying Book**
Everything® **Home Improvement Book**
Everything® **Internet Book**
Everything® **Jewish Wedding Book**
Everything® **Low-Fat High-Flavor Cookbook**
Everything® **Money Book**
Everything® **Pasta Book**
Everything® **Pregnancy Book**
Everything® **Study Book**
Everything® **Trivia Book**
Everything® **Wedding Book**
Everything® **Wedding Checklist**
Everything® **Wedding Etiquette Book**
Everything® **Wedding Organizer**
Everything® **Wedding Vows Book**
Everything® **Wine Book**

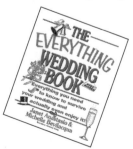
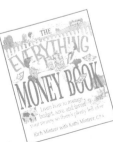
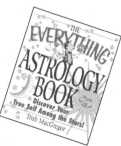
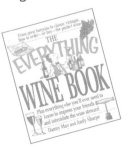
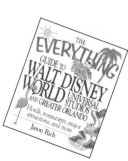